THE EYE AND THE MIND

PHILOSOPHICAL STUDIES SERIES

Founded by Wilfrid S. Sellars and Keith Lehrer

VOLUME 58

CHARLES LANDESMAN
Hunter College and the Graduate School
of the City University of New York

THE EYE AND THE MIND

Reflections on Perception and the Problem of Knowledge

SPRINGER-SCIENCE+BUSINESS MEDIA, B.V.

A C.I.P. Catalogue record for this book is available from the Library of Congress.

ISBN 978-90-481-4343-6 ISBN 978-94-017-3317-5 (eBook)
DOI 10.1007/978-94-017-3317-5

Printed on acid-free paper

CONTENTS

PREFACE

This book is a discussion of some of the major philosophical problems centering around the topic of sense perception and the foundations of human knowledge. It begins with a characterization of our common sense understanding of the role of the senses in the acquisition of belief, and it argues that scientific accounts of the processes of perception undermine salient parts of this understanding. The naive point of view of direct realism cannot be sustained in the light of a scientifically instructed understanding of perception. This critique of direct realism points to the correctness of the representative theory of perception characteristic of such early modern philosophers as Descartes and Locke, and it also endorses the subjective turn that they defended. It argues that these positions do not require introducing sense data into the picture, and thus it avoids the intractable problems that the sense datum philosophy introduces. In addition, several versions of cognitive accounts of sense perception are criticized with the result that it is unnecessary to characterize sensory processes in intentional terms.

The book then turns to a leading question introduced into modern philosophy by Descartes and Locke, the question of the accuracy of the information delivered by the senses to our faculty of belief. In particular, how accurate are our representations of the secondary qualities? The case of color is considered in detail. The view that is defended is color skepticism which says that nothing has any color, that all our judgments predicating colors of objects are false. Because this view seems so implausible on its face, a whole chapter is devoted to replying to a number of objections.

The subjective turn as propounded by Descartes led him to adopt a skeptical starting point for his epistemological reflections. This book ends with a discussion of knowledge and skepticism and argues that the subjective turn and the representative theory of perception do not inevitably lead to skepticism about the senses. In order to avoid skepticism, it is necessary to develop a proper understanding of our concept of knowledge and the relation between knowledge and justification. Skeptical arguments directed at our perceptual judgments fail to show that these judgments are not instances of knowledge.

I have attempted to write this book so that it is accessible both to philosophers who are informed about the issues it discusses and to other readers who are not. The presentation is self-contained and avoids technical jargon wherever possible. Although the aim of the book is to defend a number of philosophical views on topics pertaining to human knowledge, it is capable of serving as an introduction to these topics for the general reader.

The writing of parts of this book was supported by a PSC/CUNY research grant. A few pages from Chapter Seven were incorporated into my article "Why Nothing Has Color: Color Skepticism" that is included in *The Theory of Knowledge: Classical and Contemporary Readings*, edited by Louis P. Pojman (Belmont, California: Wadsworth Publishing Company, 1993); they are reprinted here with the permission of the editor.

This book is dedicated to my brother Bruce Landesman, a fellow philosopher and a wonderful person.

CHAPTER ONE

UNDERSTANDING VISION: COMMON SENSE VS. SCIENCE

OUR COMMON UNDERSTANDING OF VISION

Inquirers engaged in the scientific enterprise search for facts and laws in a methodical and deliberate way. Their claims to know are controlled by the requirements of empirical testing and logical reasoning. But not all our knowledge is scientific; a great deal of it consists of the casual and unmethodical acquisition of information as we go about our daily tasks. This common sense knowledge is directed not only at particular facts. We also acquire general views about things. Without a substantial stock of generalizations in our possession, we would be at a loss to know how to interpret and make sense out of the variety of particular facts that flood in upon us at every moment of our waking lives. If we think of theories as sets of generalizations used for interpretive and explanatory purposes, then we are theoreticians whether we know it or not. We find ourselves with general views, and in many cases we do not know how we have arrived at them.

Among the items in the world that are comprehended by our prescientific general understanding are our fellow human beings. A good deal of human behavior is predictable and routine; what most people do most of the time doesn't surprise or astound us; their actions fit into our established understanding of how people characteristically behave and of what motivates such behavior. If we were to formulate this general understanding in words, we would find ourselves with a rather extensive though imprecise psychological theory. This is our common sense psychology in contrast to the scientific psychology based upon explicit theory construction and empirical testing. I do not mean to imply that there is a sharp cleavage between them. It is a matter of some controversy as to the nature of their relation. But some preliminary suggestions are relevant.

Questions that arise about human behavior within the framework of our common sense understanding occasionally cannot be answered within its terms. For example, last night I had a disturbing dream the details of which I have now almost forgotten. Why did I have that dream at that time? Why are dreams that are vivid and disturbing so easily forgotten? These are very interesting questions, but I have no idea how to answer them. Our common sense psychology has nothing to say beyond the most feeble conjectures. But scientific psychology is not at a loss for words on the topic of dreams. In practice much of scientific psychology builds upon and extends our common sense understanding. Through ingenious experiments and rigorous testing, it augments our common sense knowledge of familiar topics.

Occasionally, however, theories within scientific psychology clash with their prescientific counterparts and come to replace them. This can easily be seen in those instances when a culture's views are influenced by superstition. For example, the Bible tells us in *Genesis* 40 that Joseph was capable of interpreting dreams so as to predict the future and that his predictions came true. Current theories within scientific psychology do not support the view that dreams are a reliable basis for forecasting the future. But superstitions aside, theories which claim to be scientific occasionally support interpretations of behavior that clash with those offered by our common sense understanding. For example, a person may explain why he is so angry by alleging certain deficiencies or characteristics in the objects of his anger. In contrast, a scientific psychology such as the one stimulated by Freud's researches into the unconscious may claim that such explanations are intended to conceal the person's real reasons. One consequence of the growth of depth psychology is that much of our common sense understanding of human motivation can no longer be taken at face value. I do not here mean to endorse the Freudian alternative to common sense; there are well known doubts about its adequacy. But I mention it as an illustration of how scientific theorizing may raise serious questions about the correctness of common sense explanations.

Off all the human senses, vision is the one that provides the fullest and most direct consciousness of the world. When one opens one's eyes, the objects of the world appear to us in their full glory, along with their qualities and relationships. Finding out about the world through seeing seems to be easy, uncomplicated, and unproblematic.

That we respond as we do when we look at things suggests that we have a certain general understanding of vision and how it relates us to the world that it discloses. This general understanding is our *common sense theory of vision*. Not only does it include some views about the objects that we see but also contains thoughts about our seeing of them. Thus our common sense theory includes a primitive and undeveloped psychology of vision. This common sense theory is part of our wider pre-scientific conceptual scheme that incorporates our basic concepts of interpretation as well as generalizations and information that we use in applying our concepts. This common sense theory is not something whose content is revealed just by introspection or inward consciousness; it must be abstracted from the details of our use of visual information. It is implicit and implicated in our responses to the world, in both our actions and thoughts. In what follows, I shall present and explain what I take to be some of its main tenets.

In the first place, we take seeing things to be a *direct apprehension* of them. Sometimes we acquire information indirectly, from what others tell us, for example, or by means of signs and evidence. Often we discover what must have happened by an inference from data taken as premises. In contrast, seeing something is non-inferential. When you see something, it is right there before your eyes. When I see, for example, a yellow pencil, I do not infer its existence from signs; I am inspecting the pencil itself. The belief that I acquire that there is a yellow pencil lying upon my desk is not based upon evidence; you don't need evidence when you have the very thing itself.[1] What we learn from what we see may be made the basis of an inference, but all inferences must, sooner or later, be traced back to a direct acquaintance with objects. This part of our common sense theory I shall call *the principle of direct acquaintance*.

In the second place, we take for granted that the things that we see exist independently of our seeing them. Looking and seeing are not creative activities like painting and writing that produce their own objects. In vision, we apprehend what is already there. The things we apprehend exist prior to our apprehending them and continue to exist after we look away. Some minor qualifications of this assumption are, perhaps, in order. Occasionally, an object of vision may come into existence just as we look at it and cease to exist just as we look away, a soap bubble, for instance. But this a just a coincidence; our visual actions neither created nor destroyed the bubble. In addition, in order to obtain a view of something, we may have to modify our surroundings in some way, for example, by removing something that is blocking our sight. Vision may be accompanied by various interventions in the world; we often need to act in order to see or to see better. But we do not think that seeing in abstraction from the interventions that precede and follow it is itself an intervention in the world. In seeing we are receptive; an independent reality is given to us. There is a world that we never made, and vision is one way to gain access to it. I shall call this *the principle of independent existence.*

Third, it is not only the objects we see that have independent existence but also their features. Through vision, we become acquainted not only with things but also with their colors, shapes, sizes, motions and distances. And these features are, we think, no more created and destroyed by our visual acquaintance then are the things themselves. The pencil I see really is yellow, and its color belongs to the pencil whether we see it or not.[2] In this respect these features are equal. Color is no less independent of vision than is shape. This is *the principle of feature objectivity.*

Fourth, not only are the things and their features that we see independent of our seeing them, for the most part we see them as they really are in themselves. We think that vision reveals a ready made world as it exists in itself. Occasionally, however, our eyes do mislead us. Sometimes things look different from the way they really are, and this may lead us to acquire false beliefs about them. A round plate can look elliptical when viewed from a certain angle; a straight stick in water can look bent. When there is a deviation between how something looks and how it is, the visual perception is not *veridical* in just the respect in which the deviation occurs. When there is no deviation, the perception is veridical in that respect. In some cases, there appear to be things when there is nothing there at all; consider Macbeth's hallucination of a bloody dagger. What Macbeth experienced was a failure in veridicality not merely with respect to some feature of the object but with respect to its very existence. Failures of veridicality do not always mislead. Occasionally I see a spot in front of my eyes due, I am told, to some protein particles floating about in the fluid behind my eye ball. Yet I do not believe that the world is really spotty. The spots are due to me, not to the world. But although appearances occasionally fail to match reality, we think that most of the time there is an accurate match. I shall label this *the principle of presentational accuracy.*

Fifth, we think that the world that is disclosed in vision is contemporary with our seeing it. When I observe the various items that are lying on the table on which I am writing these words, I am convinced beyond any doubt that they are on the table at the time that I am observing them. According to the principle of direct acquaintance, the world as it is seen is directly disclosed; no inference is required to obtain visual access to it. Now I am adding that the facts that are so disclosed are simultaneous with their disclosure. Call this *the principle of simultaneity.*

Sixth, we recognize that visual perception is a certain function or activity of humans and animals that can be divided into various phases. For example, suppose that I have misplaced my watch and begin to search for it. In the first phase, I look around the room; next I see the watch lying on the floor; finally I come to believe or realize that it is lying on the floor. In this example, there are three phases: the process of conducting a search with one's eyes; the seeing or catching sight of what I was searching for; and finally the acquisition of knowledge or information based upon the seeing. If the information acquired is correct or accurate, then this third phase is something of a cognitive achievement; I have learned something I did not previously know. The searching by looking is an active process extended in time in which various things come into view and which may involve moving about and other actions. The middle phase is seeing proper. The thing I am looking for has come into view; I see it. Seeing something is also something of an achievement: what I see is actually there, right before my eyes. This is not a cognitive achievement as is the third phase. It is not a learning of something new. But by seeing a watch that was actually there, my perception was veridical; there was a match between appearance and reality; and that counts as a type of achievement.[3] Usually when one says "A sees B" there is an implication that there really is something, B, that is seen. In certain cases, however, we use "see" when we are hallucinating as when we say that Macbeth sees a bloody dagger or when I say that I see spots before my eyes. Here the implication of an achievement is cancelled, and we use "see" to have the same force as "appear" or "look."

Seventh, we acknowledge that seeing something can be either qualified or unqualified. What I mean is this. There are things that are too small or too far away to see. We can, however, compensate for our frailties and limitations by the use of various instruments such as the microscope or telescope or periscope. When we use an instrument to look at something that we could not otherwise see, we can then see it, but we qualify our assertion of seeing it by saying that we saw it through a microscope or through a telescope or through a periscope. Similarly, if I saw the president deliver a speech on television, I would not say, simply, that I saw the president last night; that would be misleading; rather I would qualify my remark by saying that I saw him on television. Unqualified seeing is just seeing something with our naked eyes. In this case, we think that we are not using an instrument; we are just using our eyes. We normally do not think that our eyes are instruments like a microscope. Of course, when we learn of the complex structure of our eyes and of the various physical processes that make seeing possible, we may come to think of our eyes as instruments too. We may come to think that when we look at something through a microscope, we are using two instruments, the microscope and our eyes. But that new way of thinking about our eyes is a product of science which reveals certain analogies between the instruments that we make and our visual apparatus. It does not as such belong to our common sense theory of vision. Of course, as the results of scientific investigation become well known and become entrenched in our thought about the world, they may enter our conceptual scheme and add to it or modify it. There is no impregnable wall between science and common sense.

In the eighth place, we recognize that the visual function plays a central role in controlling and motivating our behavior. When our eyes are open and we move around, we are being continuously flooded with information about our surroundings, information that we use to avoid misadventures and to realize our goals. Vision is part of the human and animal system of feedback mechanisms that keep our movements from deviating from their intended course. It tells us about items in our environment that we may want to obtain or avoid. In our common sense psychology, vision is not just an isolated function but plays a central role in directing our behavior.[4]

Ninth, a remark is in order about the variety of items that we are able to see. Not only am I able to see the pencil when I look at it, but I am also able to perceive its color and shape; I can see how long it is and how far away it is; I can see it lying on the table, and when it rolls off the table,

I can see it falling to the floor. The items one is capable of seeing are instances of a variety of types or categories: things, qualities, relations among things, events or happenings, and states of affairs. One type of item deserves special mention because of problems it raises; these are images. For example, if you look at a bright light for a time and then turn your eyes towards a blank wall, you will very likely see an after-image floating in the space in front of you. Although our common sense conceptual scheme recognizes images as among the items that are accessible to our senses, their status is a bit ambiguous. Are they independent items like the pencil or are they subjective items like a sensation of pain? It is not evident that our common sense theory of vision contains the resources to provide a definite answer to this question.[5]

Finally, suppose we raise the question whether other animals see as we see. Do dogs see in color? Do insects perceive distances and shapes as we do? Such questions cannot be answered on the basis of casual observation. They are questions for the biologist rather than for the man on the street. But in the way that I have formulated them, I have assumed that we human beings see in the same way as one another. For instance, we think we see in color and in the same colors. Of course, we understand that some people have deficits, diseases, and abnormalities in their visual apparatus. Some people are color blind and are incapable of perceiving the normal range of colors. We have a conception of what normal vision amounts to in the human species. Even though we may easily be led to doubt that we know what it is like for a beetle to see things, we are usually in no doubt about what it is like for other people to see things. Unlike certain capacities whose presence is distributed unequally among human beings, we think that perceptual capacities are relatively uniform.

This completes my account of our common sense theory of vision. Certain parts of it have been rejected by philosophers and psychologists who have found it difficult to integrate it into the theoretical scheme of exact science. In particular, the principles of direct acquaintance, feature objectivity, and presentational accuracy are vulnerable on this score. Some philosophers, I have in mind George Berkeley and those persuaded by his immaterialist philosophy, have even rejected the realism implied by the principle of independent existence. On the other hand, there is a tradition of common sense philosophy which claims that our ordinary, everyday way of talking and thinking about perception is acceptable as it is; this tradition is committed to showing that the common sense view is internally coherent and consistent with the facts and theories about vision uncovered by exact science. In what follows, we shall examine whether and to what extent the common sense theory can hold its own. We shall find that only a portion of it survives.

SEEING STARS

Consider a distant star; call it T. Astronomers measure stellar distances by light years, the number of years it takes light to travel between heavenly bodies. Suppose T is 100 light years away from the earth; thus it took 100 years for light to travel from T to our observatories. When I observe T and make use only of our common sense perspective, I think that I am learning about its features as they are at the time of observation. This is an instance of the principle of simultaneity. But now we have available to us a scientific story according to which we are only able to see an object when light is reflected from it or transmitted from it and enters our eyes. The science of vision has been developing this story for over three centuries, filling in its details as we learn more about light, how it interacts with bodies, how it affects human eyes, how the changes thus brought about cause changes in the nervous system and brain, and how all these enable us to see. This story is not a product of casual observation but is an example of scientific theory construction at its most sophisticated.

This scientific story tends to undermine the principle of simultaneity by making it reasonable to suppose that the features of T that I am *now* observing are those that T possessed 100 years ago. Suppose that I now see T twinkle. Then the disturbance in T that I call a twinkling occurred 100 years ago. Suppose that T exploded 50 years ago and completely disintegrated. No one will learn of this disaster for another 50 years. In thus throwing doubt upon the principle of simultaneity, I am taking certain aspects of the scientific theory of vision for granted. For example, I am supposing that the information about T that I have gained by seeing it is contained in the waves of light that T emitted 100 years ago. Anything that sight tells me about T must be contained in that light; there is no other source of information. I am also assuming that the information carried by the light is 'tied' to what was happening to T at the time when the light was emitted; there is nothing in the scientific story to justify us in supposing that the information is being continuously updated once the light leaves T. Once it leaves T, there is no way that it could continue to track what is happening to T. Of course, what the light 'tells' us about T could be misinformation rather than information; it could mislead as well as inform.

Suppose the light contains a certain feature or characteristic F that depends upon some change in T. For example, if T is pulsating, then F varies in a regular way with that series of events. If T exploded, then F was produced by that explosion. If T is turning from one color to another, then the variations in F depend upon the variations in color. Following Dretske, I shall say that, in such cases, F *indicates* the change or changes C it depends upon. The fact that F is contained in the light carries the *information* that C occurred.[6]

Suppose that I now see T explode and disintegrate. As a result, I come to believe that T just exploded. This belief is partly true and partly false. It is true in that part that says that T exploded. It is false in that part that says that the explosion just occurred. The light from T contains a feature E that indicates the explosion. In order for me to arrive at this belief, my visual system must extract that information from the light. We can think of the process of forming perceptual beliefs or judgments as consisting in part of the extraction and processing of information from the features of the signal which carry information and which our visual system is sensitive to.[7] But we cannot say that we extracted any information from the light with respect to that part of the belief that is false. Misinformation is not information. In forming it, I unconsciously made use of the principle of simultaneity in supposing that what I see occurs just when I see it. Perhaps this principle functions as a rule of operation by which our visual system works; it is part of the program rather than the data. In most cases the principle functions quite well; it leads us to suppose that in looking at the objects that environ us, we are learning about events that we *now* have to cope with, where the word "now" refers to a brief period of time approximately simultaneous with our perception. We can understand how the principle of simultaneity might have been the result of natural selection working on creatures who need to learn how to cope with changes now occurring in their environments. The principle misleads in only those cases where the need to cope is less stringent. We can bring our scientific knowledge to bear to correct our natural beliefs; we replace the belief with another which says that T exploded 50 years ago.

A perceptual belief (or judgment) is formed directly from a perception and represents something about the item or items perceived. Thus, if upon seeing a red apple I come directly and immediately to believe that there is a red apple there, I have formed a perceptual belief. Such a belief is a representation which can be false as well as true, or can be partly false and partly true, or can contain misinformation as well as information, or can indicate how things stand or fail to indicate how they stand. As the example of the exploding star shows, the formation of such a belief may involve more than just the extraction of information. I shall call the process which leads to a perceptual belief and *interpretation* of the perception. The extraction of information is part of the process of interpretation. The application of general rules is another part. In addition to the information delivered by the perceptual system and the program or inherited set of general rules, the process of interpretation also makes use of concepts and beliefs already acquired by the perceiver and made part of his cognitive system. For example, I could not form the belief that the star has exploded if I did not know what a star was and what an explosion was. This is *conceptual knowledge*, and when the items that are instances of the concepts are perceptible, they include *rules of recognition* that enable the concepts to be applied in perception.

A substantial amount of what I have just described as happening when I form the belief that T just exploded and then correct it on the basis of my knowledge of the scientific story is not itself derived directly from observation or introspection. I do not observe the light travelling from T to my eyes; the light in the scientific story is not the observable light that we see but a theoretical entity whose existence is postulated in order to explain the phenomenon of sight among other things. I am not conscious of my visual apparatus being affected by light or of its 'processing' the information it contains. I am not conscious of what my brain actually does in carrying the information to the perceptual stage. In general, although I am aware of my seeing the star and of the belief that I form, I am not aware of the intervening processes of interpretation or of the utilization of background knowledge and principles in the interpretation. That there are intervening interpretive processes of the character that I have described is hypothesized in order to explain how the human mind is able to move from perception to belief. Since the belief is derived from or based upon the perception, the character of the perception and the intervening process of derivation must contribute to the character of the belief. Since there is more to the belief than what is contributed by the perception and the information in the light, other factors already present in the mind must also contribute to the character of the belief. The task of a theory of interpretation is to propose an empirically grounded and conceptually perspicuous account of the move from perception to judgment.

EXPLANATION AND JUSTIFICATION

The sketch of the process of interpretation that I have just provided is intended as no more than a suggestion of how perceptual beliefs come to be formed. The notion of explanation involved here is a familiar one. There is a certain event to be explained—the *explanandum*—which in this case is the acquisition of a certain belief; this event is the end result of a certain process or sequence of events that begins with an object reflecting or emitting light and ends at the brain or mind of the person whose eyes are stimulated by the light. The earlier events cause or bring about the later ones, and the specific causal connections are understood as instances of law-like generalizations to be established by the sciences concerned with vision and its conditions. In this particular case, the proximate cause of the belief that T exploded consists of my seeing it explode together with the activation of those items in my established cognitive repertoire relevant to interpreting the perception and extracting from it the information that constitutes the content of the belief.

If I should say to someone that T exploded, he may ask how I know it or what my reason for believing it is or what my evidence is. This is a request not just for an explanation but for a justification. My answer would naturally be: I saw it explode; that's how I know it. In giving this answer I mention one of the proximate causes of the belief. The same event that is part of the explanation is also mentioned as providing the justification. What then is the difference between explaining and justifying?

In the explanation the formation of the belief is considered as an event, and the explanation consists in discovering its causes. Whether we are content with the proximate cause or want more distant ones depends on the question to which the explanation is a response. With regard to justification, however, the event is treated not just as something which has come into existence but as a representation with a certain content that claims that some portion of the world has a certain character. If it has the character it is represented as having, then the belief is true, otherwise false. Thus one who asks for a justification wants not merely the cause of an event but a reason for supposing that the content that the event embodies is true. The context of justification of belief and judgment is one in which the interest in truth predominates. The judgment is taken as a representation with a certain content. Justification is an attempt to show that the world exemplifies the content that the judgment asserts it to exemplify.

Even though one may mention one of the causes of a belief in providing a justification, the interest is not in the cause as being a cause but in its being such as to show the belief to be true. In giving a justification, a person can only mention causes he actually knows about. It may be the case that certain neurons fire in his brain only if they were caused to fire by an exploding star. If he knew of the firing of these neurons and if he knew they are such as to indicate the exploding of the star, then that event could be cited as evidence for the truth of his judgment. But of course, he knows nothing of what is going on in his brain when he sees the star. So he could not offer that as his justification any more than he could offer the particular pattern of excitation on his retina caused by the light from T.

However, there is a difference between being able to offer a justification and being justified. One is in a position to offer a justification when one knows of those sources or bases or causes of one's belief which are such as to support the claim that the belief is true. But it is possible that one is justified even if one is not in any position to offer a justification. Suppose for example that you believe some commonplace theorem of Euclidean geometry such as that the sum of the angles of a Euclidean triangle add up to 180 degrees. Suppose you learned it years ago in school by constructing a proof of it, a proof that was sound and that convinced you and whose soundness was verified by your teacher. Suppose now, many years later, you remembered the theorem but completely forgot the proof; in fact, you forgot that you even constructed and verified the proof. But, I would argue, you still know the truth of the theorem for you came to believe it by a process which is such as to show that it is true. Of course *you* can no longer show that it is true for you have no recollection of this process. The loss of memory does not destroy your knowledge but rather destroys your capacity to argue that you do have this knowledge. If you are in a position to provide a justification, then no only do you know the truth of the theorem, but you also know that you know it. You have knowledge about your knowledge. But in order to know something, you do not have to know that you know it. You do not have to have knowledge of knowledge in order to have knowledge. If you did have to have knowledge of knowledge in order to have knowledge, then you would be entering upon an infinite regress that cannot be completed, and thus you would not have any knowledge of anything at all.

To return to the case of perception, suppose the exploding star caused an event in the perceiver's brain that would not have occurred had the star not exploded; and suppose that brain event caused him to acquire the belief that the star exploded in such a way that he would not have acquired the belief unless the star had in fact exploded. Then his belief is true and it came about by a process that guarantees its truth. That it is true is no accident. Then I think that he knows that the star exploded and does not merely believe it. Its truth is guaranteed by the occurrence of that brain event. Of course he knows nothing of the brain event, and he does not know that it guarantees the truth of his belief. He is in no position to offer the brain event as a justification. But, as we saw, being able to offer a justification is irrelevant as far as being justified and having knowledge is concerned. Being able to offer a justification is important in being able to show to others that one is justified or has knowledge. It is thus important in science and in other practices whose success depends upon the communication of information.

In the case at hand, I am able to offer a justification for my belief that T exploded. I saw it explode, and I say so. And since it is true that I saw it explode, one would suppose that not only can I offer a justification, what I offer does succeed in *being* a justification. It is a good and sufficient reason for thinking that T exploded. But why is it a reason? What is there so convincing about it? When we turn to our common sense theory of vision for an answer, we must depend primarily upon the principle of direct acquaintance and secondarily upon the principles of independent existence and of feature objectivity. In seeing the star explode, the very event of its exploding is there before my eyes; I am in a position to inspect and then represent the event itself. And that event that I am inspecting exists independently of my inspecting it. And so do the features of the star that my inspection discovers. Seeing something is an event in which the item seen is directly apprehended; it is given. That is why we think that appealing to our seeing something provides a reason for believing in the reality of what we see; for in seeing it, we are acquainted with it and thus are assured of its reality.

Once we bring the scientific story into the picture and begin to compare it to the our common sense account, our confidence in the principle of direct acquaintance is justifiably shaken. How can we be directly inspecting an event that happened 50 years ago? Moreover if seeing is part of a process of extracting information from light and if that process consists of inner events occurring in the eyes, brains, and minds of perceivers, then our belief that T exploded seems to be a response to an inner event which we interpret as indicating a fact distant in space and time. If anything is there for us to inspect, it would seem to be that phase of the perceptual process which involves consciousness; it seems as if all that is available for inspection is something inner, not the event we see. From the common sense point of view, what we interpret when we acquire a perceptual belief is the very external and independent fact that the belief represents. Interpretation in this sense consists of inspecting a fact and forming a representation of what we are inspecting. But the scientific story suggests a wholly different account of interpretation. It suggests that perception produces an inner event within the perceiver, and that this is what is interpreted. Moreover, the process of interpretation is a process of decoding what this inner event indicates about external facts. So it looks as if the process of forming a perceptual belief is or is analogous to an inference or to the formation of an hypothesis rather than being such as the principle of direct acquaintance requires. In any case, the scientific story casts doubt not only upon the relatively superficial principle of simultaneity but also upon the fundamental principle of direct acquaintance.

NOTES

1. J.L. Austin, "Other Minds," *Philosophical Papers* (Oxford: Clarendon Press, 1961), pp. 73–74.
2. Ludwig Wittgenstein, *Philosophical Investigations* (New York: The Macmillan Company, 1968). Part I, section 275.
3. Gilbert Ryle, *The Concept of Mind* (London: Hutchinson's University Library, 1952), pp. 151-152.
4. Not only in common sense but also in scientific psychology. According to John Dewey, various philosophical traditions have recognized this function of perception: "In Platonic and Aristotelian psychology....the senses as such are essentially organs of biological activity connected with the appetite." (John Dewey, "An Empirical Survey of Empiricisms," in *On Experience, Nature, and Freedom*, ed. Richard Bernstein (New York: The Liberal Arts Press, 1960), p. 76).
5. Jonathan Westphal reflects the common sense view when he asserts: "I think it is absolutely certain that afterimages do have colour (though it does not strike my ear as correct to say that they are *coloured*), and I think that only philosophers who have painted themselves into a corner in the philosophy of mind would ever have is wished to deny such a flat empirical fact." (Jonathan Westphal, *Colour: Some Philosophical Problems from Wittgenstein* (Oxford: Basil Blackwell, 1987), p. 86).
6. Fred Dretske, *Explaining Behavior: Reasons in a World of Causes* (Cambridge, Mass.: The MIT Press, 1988), pp. 54-59.
7. Irvin Rock, *The Logic of Perception* (Cambridge, Mass.: The MIT Press, 1985), Chapters I and II.

CHAPTER 2

THE SUBJECTIVE TURN AND THE PROBLEM OF TRANSPARENCY

SENSATION AND REPRESENTATION

The difficulties we have found in our common sense views of vision pertain not just to the seeing of distant objects such as stars but to all cases of seeing. Even when we observe things close up, information about them is contained in the light waves that they reflect or emit. The perceiver gains access to this information as a result of his eyes being affected by light which thereby triggers a series of inner episodes in his nervous system and brain. Observation has a quite different meaning in the scientific story than it has for common sense. The directness and immediacy by which we seem to be visually in touch with the 'external world' is, for the scientific story, just an illusion. What we call 'seeing something' is not a simple inspection of an external fact, but the production of a chain of inner events which then are interpreted in order to extract their informational content.

This understanding of the scientific story also suggests that the status and worth of observation as a foundation for our knowledge of the 'external world' must be reconsidered. The accuracy of our perceptual judgments depends upon what happens to the information as it is conveyed from objects to the brain via various physical processes. We can ask whether, in the course of the processing of this information, it is changed or modified or distorted in any way. Does the process of interpretation add any content that was not there in the physical signal? Does the physical signal carry any content that is not present in the object observed? The answers to these questions hinge on the scientific story. The extent to which sense perception delivers an accurate representation of the external world, the extent to which our cognitive maps of nature depict nature as it really is, will be revealed gradually as the scientific story unfolds.

It appears paradoxical that the scientific story tells up about the accuracy of observation when that story itself is confirmed by methods and procedures which rely in an essential way upon observation. There seems to be a circularity here. In fact, there is no insuperable difficulty as long as the new story about observation does not destroy the confirmatory value of the data upon which the story was based. We shall return to the problem of circularity later in our discussion of skepticism in the final chapter.

Philosophers of the early modern period (I have Descartes and Locke especially in mind here) were impressed by the outlines of the scientific story that was then quite new and was just beginning to win out over the older Aristotelian account of perception. They took it for granted that visual perception is an instance or form of consciousness, and therefore they came to believe that the inner episodes produced by the stimulation of the eyes are not confined to the brain and nervous system but included a mental or subjective component. Events in the brain produce a type of mental episode labelled sensation or sense experience or sense impression. The terminology might differ from thinker to thinker but the basic point was the same: seeing a physical object includes essentially the receiving of sensations caused by the action—direct or indirect—of the object upon the sense organs.

The concept of sensation that was thus introduced to represent a mental link between brain events and perceptual judgments was not intended as a novel addition to the story of perception. It was thought that the common sense story included much the same idea; after all, we speak not only about the features that we *see* things to have, but also the features that they *look* or *appear* to have. The common sense view includes the notion of sensory appearances. However, it is not obvious that the appearances of common sense are to be understood as inner episodes. For example, J.L. Austin whose account of perception is usually quite faithful to our pre-scientific intuitions writes:

> The way things look is, in general, just as much a fact about the world, just as open to public confirmation or challenge, as the way things are. I am not disclosing a fact about *myself*, but about petrol, when I say that petrol looks like water.[1]

I do not think that common sense is as unambiguous about the issue as Austin suggests. After all, the fact that things look yellow to a person with jaundice is a fact about him, not a fact about the way things are. In general, when the conditions that determine how something looks are specific to an individual, we think that how it looks is a fact about him. When the conditions apply to everyone, we do not think we are disclosing a fact about specific persons. For the early modern philosophers we are considering, these ambiguities were resolved by interpreting all appearances as sensations in the mind. That some sensations are 'public' simply means that almost everyone will receive the same type of sensation when looking at the same object under the same circumstances. All sensations are private in their intrinsic nature as inner mental events. The public-private contrast disappears and is replaced by reference to the similarities and differences among the sensations of different persons.

Because these inner sensations embody information about the external objects that cause them, they function as representations or signs of these objects and their features. Of course, the physical events in the brains and eyes of perceivers could also be said to represent the objects that cause them as we have noted. But because sensations are intrinsically conscious items, they are representations that are accessible to the perceivers themselves. When we see something, we are directly acquainted with a visual sensation and take it as a sign of the object. Because we are conscious of the sensation, we are able to reflect upon and even criticize our perceptual takings. We can wonder whether or not the beliefs that emerge from these takings are true. We can consider whether the sensations themselves are faithful and veridical representations of their objects. Thus was born *the representative theory of perception*. It is an offspring of the scientific story combined with a claim of the essential role of consciousness in perception.

THE SUBJECTIVE TURN

Descartes was one of the first philosophers to recognize that the brain is the key physical organ in controlling mental functioning. In order for information from the external world to become represented in the mind, it is necessary that it 'pass through' the brain. In order for this mentally represented information to be used to guide and control behavior, it must 'pass through' the brain in the reverse direction. The brain functions as a central switchboard whereas the mind, through its power of decision and control, functions as a chief executive officer. The question I am here interested in is how Descartes justified introducing a mental or subjective component into the scientific story of perception. How does the mind get into the picture at all?

This is Descartes' basic argument. It is a fact that our senses sometimes deceive us. This means that things sometimes appear to be different from the way they are, that our perceptions occasionally fail to be veridical, and that we thus acquire false perceptual beliefs. In some cases the deception is so extreme that nothing is as it seems. Descartes mentioned dreams as his main example of a total failure of veridicality. From the common sense standpoint, there is no major problem here about correcting our mistakes. For example, after I dream, I awake and find myself in bed; it was *just* a dream. But the common sense view is problematic. The very reasons that I have for thinking that I have been deceived are themselves based upon the senses. My senses, however, have been shown to be somewhat unreliable, and I am led to wonder why I should trust them when I try to correct their previous failures. Perhaps my finding myself in bed is itself part of my dream. What I need in order to be able to count my perceptual beliefs as cases of genuine knowledge is some criterion, some conclusive test to distinguish veridical form non-veridical perception.

Perception itself offers no such criterion. Through the senses, I learn how things appear. What I want to know is how things really are. The mind's passage from appearance to reality provides no certitude if one is confined to the content represented by the appearances. From the fact that things look a certain way, it does not follow that they are that way. The reasons for the beliefs that my senses suggest are not conclusive; they are not reasons that generate *knowledge*.

For Descartes, a number of interesting theoretical points are founded upon these meditations on our senses. First, there is his famous skepticism. We can doubt any particular perceptual judgment; we have reason to wonder whether any such judgment counts as knowledge. But since all perceptual judgments are collectively doubtful, we can even doubt the very existence of a material world, a world that out senses claim to represent. Since the beliefs that we have about our own bodies are themselves delivered via the senses, we can even doubt that we have bodies.

Perhaps I should here switch to the first person as did Descartes in his *Meditations*. I am not entitled now to speak of 'we' but only of 'I.' After all, my beliefs about the existence of others are themselves based upon my senses. With respect to what I actually know, these meditations show that I have no reason to suppose that I am not alone in the world. The only thing that I can be sure of is that I exist and that I am having certain experiences and thoughts.

According to Descartes' argument, in order for me to establish that the system of beliefs that I started with counts as knowledge or at least as justified opinion, I must bracket or put aside this very system and search for a criterion of knowledge and truth. The argument has established that such a criterion cannot itself be based upon the senses. It must be based not upon content allegedly produced by the workings of objects upon the senses, but upon materials drawn from the mind's own nature independent of sense experience. The particular twists and turns of Descartes' attempts to overcome skepticism are of no concern to us in this discussion. Subsequent philosophical commentary has failed to find his solution convincing, and I agree with its verdict. However, subsequent commentary has found his skeptical arguments of such weight that his project of overcoming skepticism became one of the chief items on the agenda of modern philosophy. The skepticism seems to be a plausible result of the subjective turn, and that is why we shall consider it in the final chapter.

In the second place, although in perception, I can reasonably doubt the reality, I cannot doubt the appearance. For example, if I look at something and am led by my senses to believe that it is green, although I cannot be sure that it is green, although I cannot know, in the absence of a criterion, that it is green, I can be sure that it looks green. This is not quite accurate. I am not really entitled to say that *it* looks green because I have bracketed the *it*. The *it* is something that I have reason to doubt. It is more accurate to say that it is as though I were seeing something green or it looks to me as though I were seeing something green. These are things I can know.

Third, Descartes interpreted such reports about the appearances as being reports about a particular subject-matter, namely certain inner sensory episodes. These sensations possess a content; one is a sensation of green, another of red, and other of heat, another of taste. The person whose sensations they are cannot be mistaken about their existence and content provided that he is attentive and alert. A person is directly acquainted with his own sensations; there is little or no room for error here. Skepticism about the external world follows from the fact that we are not directly acquainted with bodies or their properties. Our beliefs about them should properly be understood as conclusions of an inference whose premises consist of reports about our sensations together with the criterion used to distinguish veridical from non-veridical sensations. One of the consequences of the view that we can be sure of the content of our sensations whilst at the same time be in doubt about the external world is that the content must be something intrinsic to the sensation itself, something that can be discerned within it by inspection.[2]

Fourth, Descartes classified the having of a sensation or the sensing of a sensation as a type of thinking. To have a sensation of green is to have a thought of green. Of course, we can have a thought of green in the absence of the sensation, but that just means that we have two ways of thinking of green, the vivid way via the sensation which is just as if we are presented with green itself and the less vivid way of representing green in its absence.

The reason that lies behind this assimilation of sensing to thinking is that sensing, like thinking, is *of* something or is directed to something. I can first sense a green object and then think of it; my sensing and my thinking have the same content. Or so it is claimed. That characteristic of mental episodes that consists of their having a content is frequently called *intentionality*. It is said that it is in virtue of their intentionality that mental episodes are capable of functioning as representations. Even though we can doubt the truth and veridicality of our representations, we can have direct and unassailable knowledge of their intentional contents.

Fifth, a person's mental representations are accessible only from a first person point of view. He is directly acquainted with them; therefore, his access to them is privileged; he can introspect them. The only way others can know what he is thinking is by observing his behavior and by listening to what he says; their access is indirect and is not privileged in the relevant sense. This inherent lack of direct access by others means that mental representations are private.

Sixth, although, for Descartes, some of our mental representations are produced by means of brain activity, a careful study of the brain is incapable, of itself, of revealing either their existence or content. What goes on in the brain are physical events with physical properties. A study of the brain from a third person or objective view fails to reveal any intentionality whatever. As far as the objective point of view is concerned, a person is like a machine or robot with no trace of mind. Mentality, characterized by intentionality, privileged access and privacy, is made plain only via the first person point of view.[3] For Descartes, by comparing what we learn from the first and third person points of view, we come to realize that mental representations cannot plausibly be identified with brain events. Mind and body are distinct, and materialism is incorrect. It is unintelligible to suppose that the characteristic features of mentality are realized in the brain. There is nothing like mind that matter displays.

This subjective turn of Descartes', though prompted by the scientific story with its postulation of inner events, is not, strictly speaking, necessitated by it. Additional considerations are needed to argue for the presence of mental factors over and above the physical ones and to argue against the identification of the mental with physical inner episodes. Although many (though not all) of the philosophers of the early modern period accepted many aspects of Descartes' subjective turn, the main tendency of recent thought has been to reject it. His dualistic line of thought has been ridiculed by Ryle as the dogma of the ghost in the machine.[4] There are certain excesses in Descartes' thought which are not strictly justified by the arguments that have been given above, such as his view that the mind is a substance distinct from the body. But a substance dualism is not required by the subjective turn as I have recounted it; it is an additional factor that needs separate arguments. What I want to emphasize here is not the truth but the plausibility of the subjective turn. It is still a prominent item on the agenda of philosophy.

THE PROBLEM OF TRANSPARENCY

The issue raised by the subjective turn that I will now address is whether or not Descartes is correct in thinking that when we see something, there exists an inner event that consists of a visual sensation or visual experience. There are two parts to this issue. The first is the question whether visual sensations exist at all; the second is, if there are indeed visual sensations, do they have the characteristics Descartes ascribed to them such as privacy, privileged access, and intentionality. Let us start with the first.

In his famous paper, "The Refutation of Idealism," G.E. Moore noted:

> In every sensation or idea we must distinguish two elements, (1) the 'object,' or that in which one differs from another, and (2) 'consciousness,' or that which all have in common—that which makes them sensations or mental facts.[5]

Moore here thinks that in perception there is something going on that he labels "sensation." He provides a certain analysis of what a sensation is: it consists of an object together with consciousness or awareness of that object. If I see something red and then something green, I am having distinct sensations because, although the element of consciousness is the same in both, their objects differ. We should note that a sensation for Moore is not just an inner event but is a complex entity that includes both consciousness and its object. If we suppose that consciousness is something inner, then all sensations are alike in their inner constituents. Unlike Descartes' approach, sensations do not differ in their intrinsic contents; in fact there is no mention of intrinsic contents at all. Since consciousness is able to 'reach out' to an object, there is no need for intentional contents to represent an object; consciousness is not a representational function on Moore's account. In this respect, his view is faithful to our common sense understanding of vision, and it should be understood as a reaction against the subjective turn.

Moore points out what he takes to be a special feature of consciousness, its transparency:

> When we refer to introspection and try to discover what the sensation of blue is, it is very easy to suppose that we have before us only a single term. The term 'blue' is easy enough to distinguish, but the other element which I have called 'consciousness'—that which the sensation

> of blue has in common with the sensation of green—is extremely difficult to fix. That many people fail to distinguish it at all is sufficiently shown by the fact that there are materialists. And, in general, that which makes the sensation of blue a mental fact seems to escape us: it seems, if I may use a metaphor, to be transparent—we look through it and see nothing but the blue.[6]

The transparency of consciousness means that when we try to attend to our inner experiences in order to describe them, we only find their objects. Consciousness itself and its intrinsic features, if it has any, escape us. Awareness seems to lack introspectible features. Here again Moore is being faithful to our common sense understanding. As I pointed out in the first chapter, that understanding includes a principle of direct acquaintance; in visual perception, an object is directly given. When we reflect on what goes on in visual perception, we find simply an object of which were are aware. Moore takes his stand on what we find or seem to find or rather seem not to find via introspection. He takes his stand firmly on our pre-scientific understanding; he sees no need to modify this understanding by reference to the scientific story.

Although consciousness escapes introspection, Moore does not want to conclude that we have no access at all to consciousness via introspection. He just thinks that we should try harder:

> When we try to introspect the sensation of blue, all we can see is the blue: the other element is as it were diaphanous. Yet it *can* be distinguished if we look attentively enough, and if we know that there is something to look for.[7]

But there is something futile about this suggestion. If consciousness eludes introspection because it is transparent, trying harder could not succeed in bringing it into view. For it could only be brought into view to the extent that it is not transparent, to the extent that its intrinsic features, if it has any, are introspectible and are thus able to halt our march straight to the object. But because consciousness gives the object directly, there is no need for it to have any introspectible inner features. If it had any, they would get in the way of the object.

Moore's argument should be interpreted as a way of denying the full subjective turn of Descartes. Moore is not a materialist; consciousness is not a physical event. But mentality is a very simple affair on his view. Whereas Descartes and Locke subjectivized the secondary qualities such as color and sound because the scientific story appeared to find no room for them in the physical world, Moore attempts to re-objectivize them by insisting that they belong to objects, not to consciousness. Moore's standing firm on the common sense understanding presupposes that the scientific story must be so interpreted as to be consistent with that understanding. However, there is a tension in his view because he recognizes that common sense methods such as introspection have difficulty in verifying that understanding. This is a tension not only in Moore's thought, but also in our common sense understanding itself.

SKEPTICISM ABOUT CONSCIOUSNESS

If consciousness eludes introspection and if trying harder won't help, how can we be sure that there is anything that the term "consciousness" stands for? If consciousness is transparent, then it is featureless; if it is featureless, it is unobservable and thus lacks standing in both the common sense and scientific accounts of perception. Here is an opening for a skeptic to wonder whether we have any need for the concept of consciousness at all, at least in the way that Moore understood it. William James stated the point quite precisely when he wrote: "I believe that 'consciousness,' when once it has evaporated to this estate of pure diaphaneity, is on the point of disappearing altogether."[8] Perhaps the better way is to just drop talk of consciousness and replace it with reference to our overt and covert behavioral responses to objects.[9] We could then avoid the subjective turn, drop the story of inner mental episodes and intentional contents, and become straight out materialists.

But before taking this route, we should try to understand why Moore and others were led to suppose that there is such a thing as consciousness in the first place. Perhaps the following explanation will suffice. Consider a conceptual fact of the sort represented by "John sees a green book." If we are guided by the sentence in which we represent this fact, we can argue that the fact has a certain structure which includes as its constituents or parts the person who sees, the object that is seen and a relation between them indicated by the perceptual verb. Perceptual verbs appear to stand for relations between persons and objects. There are a variety of perceptual verbs such as "see" and "hear." When we speak of someone's hearing something, we are asserting a relation between him and a sound; when we speak of his seeing something, we are asserting a relation between him and a colored object. When the objects differ, we use different perceptual verbs, but the relation is always the same. Moore selects "consciousness" as the name of that relation which stays the same in all perceptual acts although its object varies. Thus Moore's view seems motivated by two factors: one is the relational structure of the sentences we use to describe our perceptions; another is an assumption that differences in perceptual verbs can be explained by reference to type differences among their objects and that what makes them all *perceptual* verbs is the constant element of consciousness. However, there is another account of the relational structure of these sentences that avoids the assumption of consciousness without committing us to the subjective turn. Before we turn to it, I need to make some remarks about the nature of belief.

BELIEF AND JUDGMENT

Thus far I have used the terms "belief" and "judgment" interchangeably. It is now time to distinguish them. By a judgment I mean an act of asserting the truth (or falsehood) of some proposition or of accepting (or denying) its truth or falsehood. Judging is something that we do. When, for example, I look around the room for my spectacles and suddenly recognize them as being on the mantle, that is a judgment; I am mentally asserting: "There are my spectacles." A judgment is an event that occurs at a particular time. The formulation of a judgment in words is the making of a statement and its product is the statement made. But words are not the only medium in which a judgment can be made. If I ask someone where my spectacles are, he may, instead of stating that they are on the mantle, draw a picture of them lying on the mantle. Judgments can be made of oneself or to others, in speech or in writing or in some other symbolic medium.

A judgment frequently gives rise to a belief. After recognizing my spectacles on the mantle, I come to believe that they were there all the time while I was looking for them. A belief is not an event or episode but a state of the believer that can last for a long period of time. It can persist even when one is not thinking of it. It is not an act like a judgment but a state or condition capable of persisting indefinitely, although it can gradually fade away and be forgotten. A belief and judgment may have the same propositional content. What I judge to be true at one time, I may also believe to be true for a much longer period of time. Both beliefs and judgments are capable of being cases of knowledge of the propositions judged and believed to be true. Thus both the judgment that my spectacles are on the mantle as well as the belief that is acquired as a result of the judgment are examples of my knowing where my spectacles are.[10]

What kind of state is a belief? The most common view is that it is a disposition, and among those who hold this view, the most common account of what sort of disposition it is is that it is a behavioral disposition. A disposition is a power or capacity or liability in an object to produce a certain result. Thus the fragility of a vase is its liability to break easily when dropped or struck. We say: "If it were to be dropped or struck, it would very likely break." The counter-factual conditional sentence is usually taken as the standard way of representing a disposition. The reason in favor of the dispositional theory is that people use their beliefs to guide their behavior; it is a short but, I think, mistaken step to conclude that having the capacity to guide behavior is the essential nature of belief.

Even if beliefs were dispositions, the behavioral theory is far too narrow. After all, my beliefs control my subsequent thoughts, reasonings, feelings, and emotions as well as my subsequent peripheral behavior. But the dispositional theory, even if it were broadened to include mental as well as behavioral consequences, would constitute a confusion of what beliefs characteristically do with what beliefs are. When a person acquires a belief, he thereby acquires certain information (or misinformation) about a determinate subject matter. A belief is a state of a person in which that information is stored. To have the belief that such and such is the case is to possess the information (or misinformation) that such and such is the case. Because we frequently say of information that we have stored and have available to us that we remember it, I shall classify belief states as memory states. Memory states are, of course, useful to us, and certain kinds of information are indispensable to our survival and well being. It is very likely that the survival of certain animal species including the human species depends upon their capacity to store information as beliefs. We can, reasonably, speak of the biological functions of beliefs. Such functional characterizations tell us what creatures capable of storing information are capable of doing with it. But that does not mean that the states which make it possible to accomplish these results are nothing more than states which make it possible to accomplish these results. Beliefs are essentially memory states and contingently functional states. Of course, in virtue of having beliefs, certain contrary to fact conditionals are true of the creatures that have them. In that respect, beliefs have a dispositional character. But that is true of any sort of state, not just beliefs. There is nothing uniquely dispositional about beliefs.

Sometimes when a person acquires information or learns something new, he stores it not in his brain but elsewhere, in a notebook or in a diary or on a computer disk. We do not always trust our memories or think that we have enough storage space in our brain to hold all the information we need. Suppose I have recorded some fact F in my notebook, and someone asks whether I believe in the existence of F. I check my notebook and answer that I do. Originally when the human race acquired the concept of belief, the most common site of information storage was within the person himself, and so we became accustomed to think of beliefs as states of persons. But if we think of beliefs more generally as stored information and think of sites of storage as any places to which we have access, then we need not think of our beliefs as states of ourselves but of states of anything to which we have access in which we have stored information that we accept. Books, libraries, disks, etc. are in almost a literal sense extensions of the information storage capacities of our brains. Thus we are no longer restricted to a biological concept of belief.[11]

Let me focus attention now on the narrower biological concept of belief as a state of humans and animals. There are certain arguments against the identification of beliefs with such memory states, most of which are based upon what we do when we communicate our beliefs to others. For example, when I say to someone that I believe P, I am usually not reporting an inner state but rather asserting P. When someone asks me whether or not I believe P, I do not search my memory but consider whether or not I have good reasons for asserting P. So it does not look as if ascriptions of belief are ascriptions of inner states of persons.[12]

These considerations are, however, too weak to overthrow the identification of beliefs with states. Suppose that I have already learned P, I am not in doubt of it, and I am asked whether I believe it. I reply: "I believe that P." One of the things that I am doing in producing this speech act is to communicate my acceptance of P to my auditor. By implication I am also communicating that I am willing to assert P and thus take on responsibility for its being true. But my reply is founded on the fact that I have already learned that P and that I am in possession of that information. And that is all that is claimed in asserting that beliefs are memory states. Exactly how and where the information is stored is a biological question not resolved by noting that our concept of belief is the concept of a state in which information is stored.

If I have not already learned P, if I have no view about it, and I am asked whether or not I believe it, then, of course, it would be useless to survey my memory states to answer it. The question would then be interpreted to be asking whether or not I should accept P, whether or not I should place it in the site of accepted information, and the only way to answer it would be to survey the reasons and evidence for and against P. In general, speech acts in which we report certain facts may also perform certain other communicative functions simultaneously; these latter functions do not cancel the fact reporting function but frequently presuppose it.

NOTES

1. J. L. Austin, *Sense and Sensibilia* (Oxford: Clarendon Press, 1962), p. 43.
2. Here is how Edmund Husserl puts the point: "In the perception, in the experiences of consciousness themselves, that of which we are conscious is included *as such*—...the perception is *in itself* a perception of something, of 'this tree.'" *The Crisis of European Sciences and Transcendental Phenomenology* (Evanston: Northwestern University Press, 1970), p. 85.
3. This formulation of Descartes' view owes a great deal to Thomas Nagel's "What is it like to be a bat?" in his *Mortal Questions* (London: Cambridge University Press, 1979), pp. 165-180.
4. Gilbert Ryle, *The Concept of Mind* (London: Hutchinson's University Library, 1952), Chapter One.
5. G. E. Moore, *Philosophical Studies* (London: Routledge and Kegan Paul, 1922), p. 20.

6. *Ibid.*, p. 25.
7. *Ibid.*
8. William James, "Does 'Consciousness' Exist?" in *Essays in Radical Empiricism and a Pluralistic Universe* (New York: E. P. Dutton and Co., 1971), p. 4.
9. For this move see B.A. Farrell, "Experience" in V.C. Chappell (ed.), *The Philosophy of Mind* (Englewood Cliffs, New Jersey: Prentice Hall, 1962).
10. In some recent discussions, a distinction is made between an occurrent and a dispositional sense of "belief," and what I have classified as judgment is assimilated to the occurrent sense. But as the following paragraphs make clear, I am skeptical whether there is a dispositional sense, and I do not think that datable acts of judgment are properly classified as beliefs.
11. For a further discussion of an 'objective' conception of belief and knowledge, see Karl Popper's "Epistemology without a Knowing Subject," in his *Objective Knowledge: An Evolutionary Approach* (Oxford: Clarendon Press, 1973). I make a few further remarks about this 'objective' conception in Chapter Eight.
12. For a battery of arguments against identifying beliefs with states of persons, see Chapter Two of Arthur collins' *The Nature of Mental Things* (Notre Dame, Indiana: University of Notre Dame Press, 1987).

CHAPTER 3

COGNITIVE THEORIES OF SENSATION AND PERCEPTION: A CRITIQUE

THOUGHT AND VISION

If one rejects the reality of consciousness as Moore understands it, there remains the need to replace his account of perception with a better one. How shall one understand propositions of the form "x sees y" without bringing consciousness into the picture? And since this form suggests that seeing is a relation, is there some alternative analysis which preserves its relational structure? Here is a suggestion of D.M. Armstrong's: "Perception...is the acquiring knowledge of, or inclination to believe in, particular facts about the physical world, by means of our senses."[1] this is one way of developing Descartes' view that sensing is a kind of thinking. We see something when we are having veridical visual sensations; a visual sensation is just the acquiring of a belief or an inclination to believe; it is veridical when the belief is true; that is what veridicality consists of. When a veridical sensation is acquired by means of the stimulation of the visual system by light reflected by or emitted from an object, then we see it. Since the sensation is the acquiring of a true belief caused by the object of that belief, we have knowledge as well. Since seeing includes a causal relation between the perceiver and the object, the relational structure of seeing is preserved. Seeing something in particular and sense perception in general are interpreted in this account as cognitive achievements. For this reason, I shall label this type of view *the cognitive theory of perception*. The version of the cognitive theory that we are now considering is the one which assimilates sensing to believing.

This version cannot, I think, be true. In the first place, we see many more things than we can ever form beliefs about. Just consider the enormous number of items that are capable of occupying a person's field of vision at any one time and compare that to the rather restricted number of beliefs that he is capable of acquiring about just some of them. Usually we acquire beliefs and make judgments only about those items we notice or pay attention to or are at the center of the visual field or are of interest to us. It is as if there is a filter that stands between the visual system and the belief formation system of the mind that allows only some information to enter. We can speculate that the function of the filter is to allow only useful information to be stored in order to avoid overloading the system. Perhaps pressures of natural selection have allowed the survival of organisms with such a filter.

A second difficulty is that although there is always a tendency for perception to produce judgment and belief, nevertheless, perception can occur without thought. Suppose one looks at a painting that one has never seen before. At first one is flooded with information about its visual content. In a brief time, one acquires an enormous number of beliefs. Suppose, now, one continues to look at it for pleasure rather than information; as time passes, the stream of information diminishes although the painting remains in full view. We can suppose the stream to wither away as we continue to look at it. Of course, other thoughts may occur; the painting may suggest many things in one's past experience; but these associations are no part of one's seeing the painting; they are not bits of information that one receives from the object in view. Not only can we suppose that at a limit seeing can occur without belief acquisition but that seeing can remain the same whole the beliefs acquired can vary. These facts imply that contrary to the theory, our concept of perception does not incorporate the concept of belief acquisition. The relation between these two concepts is a contingent one even though being a source of information is clearly a major biological function of perception.

There is another version of the cognitive theory that does not assimilate sensing to believing, but distinguishes between them. It claims, however, that sense perception consists of the interpretation of our sensations whose product is a judgment or belief. It is common for accounts of perception to claim that sense perception essentially involves an inferential component whose conclusion is a judgment.[2] An object is given in a fragmentary or incomplete way via our sensations; we try to figure out or infer what is really there; the result is a belief inferred from the sensation. For example, suppose I see a tomato. What is actually given in sensation is a red, roundish, bulgy surface. This is not yet a tomato. In order for me to perceive the tomato, I must recognize that it has a part of its surface not in my field of view, that it has an inside as well as an outside, that if i were to bite into it, I should experience a certain familiar taste, and so forth. Seeing a tomato consists in inferring it from the sparse information that the senses provide. Descartes provides another example. He imagines himself looking out the window at men crossing the street. "But what do I see over and above the hats and clothing? Could not robots be concealed under these things? But I judge them to be men; thus what I believed I had seen with my eyes, I actually comprehend with nothing but the faculty of judgment which is in my mind." And shortly after, he concludes that "bodies are not, properly speaking, perceived by the senses or by the faculty of imagination, but only by the intellect..."[3]

Because this version of the cognitive theory claims with the first that there is a conceptual connection between perception and thought, it too is vulnerable to the two criticisms already provided. In addition, both accounts are based upon a deep confusion between seeing something and seeing that such and such is so and so. Let us turn to this issue.

SEEING AND SEEING THAT

If, as the cognitive theory asserts, belief and judgment are not merely characteristic products of perception but are constitutive of it, then seeing something is just a case of seeing that something is so and so. Seeing is essentially propositional in nature. In general, a statement of the form "x sees y" where "y" is to be replaced by a name or description of an object, event, quality, or state of affairs that is in sight is a report of a visual perception. We also use statements of the form "x sees that p" where "p" is replaceable by a sentence of the statement making variety. The cognitive theory is committed to the view that statements of the first type are expandable into statements of the second; this is the linguistic side of the claim that all seeing is propositional in nature.

However, the expansion cannot be carried out; statements of the "x sees y" variety do not imply nor are they implied by statements of the "x sees that p" variety. These statements have quite distinctive functions and truth conditions. In general, *sees that* statements are used to say what a person realizes or has found out or discovered. "I now see (realize, recognize) that acquired characteristics are not inherited," may be said by someone who has just been informed of Weismann's experiments. Of course, one way of finding something out is by seeing it, and in those cases one may also use a *sees that* statement to report the information that has been extracted from the visual perception. Consider "I see that *Appearance and Reality* was written by Bradley" said upon seeing a copy of that book and seeing Bradley's name written upon it. But *sees that* statements are not restricted to such contexts; they have no essential relation to visual perception.

In general, *seeing that* is a cognitive achievement. It is a case of *knowing that*. But plain and simple seeing is not a cognitive achievement; that one has something in sight does not imply that one knows anything about it.[4] Even when *seeing that* is based upon simple seeing, it is a mistake to suppose that it itself is a type of seeing. It isn't as if there are two kinds of seeing, the plain and simple variety and *seeing that*. They are not species of the same genus. It is just a linguistic accident rather than a conceptual resemblance that the word "see" is used in both cases. Perhaps the "sees that" locution originated as a metaphor in the speech of our ancestors who imagined that coming to know something is related to the soul as seeing something is related to the body.

The claim of the cognitive theory is encouraged by a peculiarity of first person reports of visual perception. When Erica says: "I see a copy of Bradley's *Appearance and Reality* on your table" we are entitled to infer that she sees that or knows that there is a copy of this book written by that author on the table. The statement in itself does not imply this. For when Peter says what Erica says by saying "Erica sees a copy of Bradley's *Appearance and Reality* on the table" his statement implies nothing about what Erica learned when she had the book in view. (Of course, given certain natural assumptions, it is reasonable to suppose that she learned certain things.) But when Erica says it, we can infer that she has knowledge because she could not have described what she saw in this way unless she had acquired this information about the book. A persons' ability to apply certain descriptions correctly and with support frequently presuppose that she has learned something or knows something even though the statements incorporating these descriptions do not entail it. The inference to Erica's cognitive achievement is not founded on her statement but on the fact that her making it depends upon her being able to produce a sentence that she would not have been able to produce without it.

Once we have distinguished between seeing and seeing that and realized that visual sensing is distinct from believing and knowing, we no longer have reason to suppose that there is any strong conceptual connection between seeing and believing. But what are we to make of the arguments provided by Descartes and many others that in seeing something we characteristically 'go beyond' what is given? Doesn't this 'going beyond' incorporate inference and judgment? And if it does, doesn't this imply that seeing, plain and simple seeing, is a cognitive achievement?

The advocates of this inference theory are correct in claiming that when we see, for example, a tomato, we see only the part of it that is facing us; there's a lot more to the tomato than its facing surface. But it is a fact about our concept of seeing that it is not necessary to see all the parts of a thing simultaneously (something that is impossible anyway) in order to see the thing. I see the tomato just by having its facing surface in view. Of course, in order for me to recognize what I see as a tomato, that is, in order for me to *see that* it is a tomato that I see, I must know that there is more to what I see than just that facing surface. So the deployment of background information and the making of inferences are usually involved in the interpretation of what I see, that is, in the act of mind in which I extract information from what I see. But this fact about the characteristic accompaniments and products of perception is not itself a fact about the very nature of perception.

LOOKING AND SEEING

There is another formulation of the cognitive theory that I want to consider, but in order to make it plausible, I need first to show that when someone sees something, that thing looks or appears in some way to her. In short, seeing entails looking. For example, when I look at and catch sight of a green cucumber, it appears in some way to me; it need not look green; it need not even look like a cucumber. But if it doesn't look in some way or other, then I haven't seen it. Seeing something involves more than just being sensitive to light waves; we could build a machine that responds differentially to light waves, but it would not be true that it sees anything. The difference between sense perception and mere sensitivity to stimuli is that the former necessarily incorporates sense experience which, within the common sense framework, is reported in appearance talk using such verbs as "looks," "sounds," "tastes," "feels," and so forth.

The new formulation of the cognitive theory relies upon the fact that appearance talk frequently brings propositions into the picture either explicitly or implicitly. "That looks to me to be green" brings in the proposition that it is green. So sense experience incorporates propositions, it is argued. How does it do so? On this formulation it does so because sense experience itself is nothing but a belief in that proposition or perhaps just a weak or hesitant belief or even just an inclination to believe. When I see a green cucumber that looks green, then, necessarily, I am in a state of mind that is inclined in the direction of judging or accepting or believing that it is green. Such a state of mind frequently fails to flower into full belief, but it is at the very least an incipient though perhaps inhibited tendency to move toward full belief, a tendency whose full development may be thwarted by opposing psychic forces. The cucumber may look blue to me, but since I already believe that it is green, my inclination to think it is blue is suppressed by my stronger conviction.

Because propositional attitudes characteristically accompany our sense experiences and are strongly bound to them by psychological and epistemological ties, one may be inclined to accept this formulation of the cognitive theory as providing an explanation for the existence of the firm ties. This formulation may also be accepted on grounds of theoretical economy: since we have to accept anyhow that there are propositional attitudes, then the reduction of sensations to attitudes means that we don't have two separate mind-body problems but only one. In addition, appearance talk is frequently used to express hesitant belief. If I look at something in circumstances in which I have difficulty making out its color, instead of saying "It's green," I will express my uncertainty by saying, "It looks green."

In addition to the reasons provided earlier against the cognitive theory which apply to this formulation as well, there are several other reasons for not accepting it. First of all, it is not consistent with the concept of appearance that is reflected in the way we attempt to justify our perceptual judgments. Suppose, upon looking at something, I say that I am inclined to believe that it is blue. One can ask for my reasons for thinking this. It is conceptually permitted that my reason is that it looks blue; that is why I hesitantly affirm it. But if appearances were themselves just hesitant beliefs, the reason that I give could not function as a reason for it would just be a report of the very belief whose reason was being requested. There is no redundancy or repetition in saying that it looks blue when asked for my reason for thinking it is blue. That it looks blue is a different, logically independent state of affairs from my being inclined to believe that it is blue. As far as I can see, the state of affairs of its looking blue includes no proposition at all among its constituents. Of course in uttering the sentence "It looks blue" I am suggesting the proposition that it is blue. But the fact that a proposition is suggested does not entail that it is part of the state of affairs asserted.

This conceptual point leads to a very fundamental epistemological issue. It is part of our conceptual scheme that we justify some of our propositional attitudes by appealing to states of affairs that are not themselves propositional attitudes. Not all justification moves within the circle of our beliefs as the coherence theory of justification claims. The reason why it does not is quite evident. If the coherence theory were correct, then our system of beliefs would be an arbitrary construction whose truth would be forever in doubt. It is part of both of our common sense picture and the scientific story that we are in contact with the 'external' world via our senses, and that our system of beliefs is not an arbitrary construction but is founded in a way that tends toward the truth. My beliefs are constrained by factors that are not beliefs, factors which also lead us to suppose that our beliefs are frequently true. But more of this later.

But why then, one might ask, are appearance statements so often used to express hesitant beliefs or belief tendencies? The main point to note is that this use is for the most part restricted to the first person. In the first person, when someone says: "I see a green cucumber," he is also intending to communicate that he knows that there is a green cucumber there. But if he is unsure of its color because of, say, a dim light or distance from the object, he would not claim to know that it is green; he would want to say something weaker. And if he knew how the object looked, he could state how it looked and simultaneously impart how he thinks it is. It is in virtue of his making the weaker statement about the appearances rather than the stronger one about what he sees that he communicates his uncertainty.

A final argument against this version of the cognitive theory is that one can acquire belief inclinations as a result of sensory stimulation without anything looking in any way. Consider a blind man equipped with machinery that determines the frequencies of light waves plus a knowledge of which colors are likely to correlate with which frequencies. He may, then, be inclined to think that the cucumber at which he is directing his light detector is green; perhaps he unsure because the frequency registered is on the border between green and blue. So he has a belief inclination produced through his sense of touch, but, being blind, nothing looks to him in any way whatever. So the attempt to reduce sense experience to beliefs or belief inclinations or tendencies has no hope of success.

SENSATIONS AND MEANING

Even though attempts to reduce sensations to a form of belief, incipient or fully explicit, are not plausible, there is another line of thinking that claims that they possess content in their own right. The basic idea stems from the representational approach to sense perception found in Descartes and Locke. I noted earlier that for Descartes, sensing is a form of thinking. Locke classifies sensation as a mode of thought: "*Sensation*...is, as it were, the actual entrance of any *Idea* into the Understanding by the Senses."[5] According to this view, when I have a sensation of red, I am having an idea and hence a thought of red. Like belief and the other propositional attitudes, a sensation has meaning or intentionality or semantic content. It is directed to an object, and thus it is a vehicle by which we become aware of objects.

By classifying sensations as ideas, Locke is suggesting that their objects are either particulars or properties. Other views claim instead that their objects are states of affairs, items representable by means of propositions. Here is one formulation of the view:

> Seeing something as red is the sort of thing that can be illusory or veridical, hence the sort of thing that has truth-conditions, and hence the sort of thing that has content. The content of this experience is that the object in question is red; and so the experience represents an object as

> having a property, about which we can legitimately ask whether it is a property that objects so represented really tend to have.[6]

The argument appears to be this. Suppose that in looking at something, I see it as red. I have, let us assume, a sensation of red. Now the object may or may not be red. My perception may or may not be veridical. To say it is veridical, according to this argument, implies that it has truth conditions that are satisfied. Also, its being non-veridical implies that it has truth conditions that fail to be satisfied. Its having truth conditions make it something like a propositional attitude such as belief. So we can say that sensations possess propositional content. An advantage of this account is that it enables us to explain how sensations manage to represent the world; they are able to perform a representational function because they possess meaning. Another advantage is that it explains how sensations carry the information that is extracted from them in the process of forming a perceptual judgment; a sensation can carry the information that the object is red in virtue of its possessing the propositional content that it is red.

There is, however, a major ambiguity in the claim that sensations possess propositional content. Smoke indicates or is a sign of fire and hence may be said to contain the information that there is a fire going on. It contains this information because of the fact that the existence of smoke depends on the existence of fire; it is an effect of the fire. A person who knows that fire causes smoke and who now observes some smoke is entitled to infer that there is a fire going on; to say that smoke in general is a sign of fire just means that because of the dependency of smoke on fire, smoke is capable of functioning to inform those capable of knowing about it of the presence of fire. If I didn't know that fire caused smoke, then smoke would not mean fire for me; it would not carry that information to me.[7] Because of the fact that the representational function of smoke with respect to fire is founded upon a contingent relation between the two, the meaning that smoke has, the sort of intentionality it possess, is extrinsic. So the claim that sensations possess propositional content may just mean that they possess extrinsic meaning or intentionality.

I suspect, however, that those who stress the analogy between sensation and belief would not be satisfied with extrinsic intentionality. There does not seem to be any general dependency relations between beliefs and the states of affairs they mean or represent. When someone believes that Columbus discovered America in 1503, he belief is false; there is no actual state of affairs represented by his belief; his belief is not a sign of anything in the sense that smoke is a sign of fire. The information (or misinformation) 'contained' in his state of mind is not based upon any dependency relation between the belief and the fact represented; there is no fact represented. So, one might argue, the sort of intentionality possessed by beliefs and other propositional attitudes is intrinsic, not extrinsic.[8] Because sensations may fail to be veridical, they are similar to beliefs; there may be no actual state of affairs represented; what they mean may fail to be realized in the world. So their intentionality is intrinsic as well. The semantic content of a sensation is part of its very nature or essence, not something connected to it from without. I think this view is incorrect. Let us consider it further.

PERCEIVING AND INFERRING

Earlier I criticized a version of the cognitive theory which says that perception consists of inferring a conclusion from our sensations, that sense perception is an inference-like process of interpretation. I mentioned in that discussion that this view confuses perception and thought, that the formation of the perceptual judgment is frequently inference-like, but it does not follow that the perception itself is inference-like. There is another view according to which the sensation itself is a product of inference. The process of forming a sensation or percept is likened to the testing of hypotheses or the solving of problems. A sensation itself, then, is something like the conclusion of a process analogous to thinking.[9] Such a view of perception may well give comfort to those who claim that our sensations possess intrinsic intentionality for it suggests that in so far as our sensations 'contain' information that is extracted and represented in perceptual judgments, they embody or exemplify propositions. The judgment is merely an explicit formulation of the proposition exemplified by the percept.

This hypothesis testing view of perception may be viewed as part of a broader constructional view according to which our sensory fields, the phenomena we are directly acquainted with, are themselves an account or picture of the external world, the world as it is in itself, and this account may not be entirely accurate. Sense perception is a process of constructing a theory about the world; the sensory manifolds that are produced may be likened to statements of the theory. Sensory fields represent the world to us; perceptual judgments are merely explicit propositional carriers of information that is already embodied in the fields. How else can sensation make information available to the organism?

There is a wonderful passage in William James' *Principles of Psychology* that provides a good starting point for discussing a constructional approach:

> What are our very senses themselves but organs of selection? Out of the infinite chaos of movements, of which physics teaches us that the outer world consists, each sense-organ picks out those which fall within certain limits of velocity. To these it responds, but ignores the rest as completely as if they did not exist. It thus accentuates particular movements in a manner for which objectively there seems no valid ground; for, as Lange says, there is no reason whatever to think that the gap in Nature between the highest sound-waves and the lowest heat-waves is an abrupt break like that of our sensations; or that the difference between violet and ultra-violet rays has anything like the objective importance subjectively represented by that between light and darkness. Out of what is in itself an undistinguishable, swarming *continuum*, devoid of distinction or emphasis, our senses make for us, by attending to this motion and ignoring that, a world full of contrasts, f sharp accents, of abrupt changes, of picturesque light and shade.[10]

By responding to some stimuli and not others, our senses function like filters keeping some information out and allowing other information to pass through. In addition, by constructing sensory manifolds with sharp contrasts, much of the information that gets through is really misinformation. When we compare the constructed world with the picture that physics provides of nature as it is in itself, we find that the correspondence between the two is quite inexact. The constructed world may register information in a manner that is useful to active organisms, but its utility does not depend upon its veridicality. The world as it appears to us is a human construct, good enough to help the human organism to survive in a perilous environment but inaccurate from the standpoint of exact representation and precise matching.

But there is as yet no room in the account that James' provides for introducing the notion of hypothesis testing. The items in the sensory manifolds are related to energies impinging upon our sense organs as effects to causes. The fact that one color is produced by a certain range of light waves and a distinct and contrasting color by another range continuous with the first is compatible with the fact that the colors are distinct effects of separate though blending ranges. It is just a case of small changes having big consequences, of small differences in quantity causing effects that differ in quality.

One place that the hypothesis testing view seems plausible is in explaining the perception of ambiguous figures. consider the duck-rabbit figure made famous by Wittgenstein's discussion in his *Philosophical Investigations*.[11] At one time it looks like a drawing of a duck and at another of a rabbit. This cannot be understood just as a difference in judgment; the judgments follow upon the perception; we say "That's now a rabbit" and then "That's now a duck" because it first looks like rabbit and then looks like a duck. The argument is that the different perceptions cannot be understood just as effects of a stimulus because the stimulus is the same in both cases.[12] Instead the sense-datum functions as an hypothesis to explain which animal figure the stimulus best approximates. Since the stimulus approximates both figures, the gestalt switch in the appearances represents a switch in hypotheses; it is as if, when the ambiguity in the figure is transmitted to the stimulus, the visual system cannot 'make up its mind', and so moves from one conclusion to another. "The 'duck' and the 'rabbit' are, on this view, alternative hypotheses. They are hypotheses roughly equally tenable on the available data: Wittgenstein's tangle of lines. Normally perception is not ambiguous in this way because there is generally sufficient evidence over any alternative hypothesis."[13]

In response to Gregory's presentation of the hypothesis testing view, Anscombe claims that an hypothesis is something that is answerable to evidence or data. But what is the evidence? Where are the data? "Input is not the same thing as evidence to which hypothesis is answerable....For *we* who perceive don't know what the input is."[14] Not only is there a problem about the evidence, there is also a problem about the agent. Who or what is forming the hypothesis and evaluating it with respect to the evidence?

Gregory replies by denying that the use of evidence is something that is essentially accessible to consciousness. "Perceptions are answerable to data much as scientific hypotheses are answerable to data. We can say that both are judged essentially by their successes and failures at prediction."[15] A percept that fails to be veridical may lead to expectations of other percepts that never arrive. Since consciousness is not indispensable, there is no difficulty in answering the question about he agent. "The 'framer' I regard as brain mechanisms, accepting current sensory data and storing past data, mainly as generalizations, generally arriving at a good bet as to what is before us, in space and time. Surely we do not *have* to say that total human beings alone have the prerogative to frame hypotheses."[16]

I am inclined to accept certain aspects of the constructional approach, particularly as characterized by James. But I have doubts about the hypothesis testing analogy.

SENSATIONS AND HYPOTHESES

That there are certain analogies between the production of sensations and the formation of hypotheses based on data does not, of course, entail that sensations are hypotheses or that they actually embody propositional content. That the visual system acts in some respects *as if* it is testing hypotheses does not imply that it really is testing hypotheses. So the hypothesis testing analogy does not really support the view that sensations possess meaning, intrinsic or extrinsic.

When we speak of forming an hypothesis on the basis of the data available, of rejecting other alternative hypotheses, of considering evidence, of further testing, of predicting future experiences, and so forth, we are not using the language of blind causation but are speaking of deliberate, controlled and controllable intellectual processes. But the way in which sensations are produced is best represented in the language of blind causation. This is much clearer, I think, when we focus on senses other than sight. The sensation of pain that I feel in my fingers when I touch a hot stove is not the result of any calculation on my part, nor is the taste sensation I receive when I chew on a slice of tomato. Because I know how heat feels and how tomatoes taste, these sensations are capable of functioning for me as signs of external facts.

But even the visual case is problematic. Let us take another look at the duck-rabbit example. The argument is that because the stimulus is the same whether we see a duck or a rabbit, the occurrence of, say, the duck appearance cannot be explained in terms of the language of blind causation but rather suggests that its occurrence is the result of some intellectual process in which the visual system is trying to figure out what is really there. First of all, it is doubtful whether the stimulus is really the same in both cases. Of course, the picture is the same, but the notion of a stimulus is ambiguous. It could refer to the distal stimulus, in this case the picture, or it could refer to certain of the effects of the picture upon the visual system. In the latter case, the retinal image could count as a stimulus, and it is by no means obvious that this is the same in both cases. When I look at the picture, I see the duck when my eyes are focused upon the duck's bill, and I see the rabbit when I attend to the area from the rabbit's eye to its mouth. In order to switch back and forth, I need to move my eyes slightly, and thus the images produced occupy a slightly different part of the retina. Thus there is a difference in stimulus that actually causes a difference in sensation. The argument for the hypothesis testing view based upon ambiguous figures collapses; it is always plausible in such cases to look for a difference in stimulus that blindly causes the sensation to occur.

That the hypothesis testing view is based upon illegitimately extending an analogy can be seen by considering the case of simple pocket calculator. The designers of the calculator have so arranged it that the blind causal processes that occur within it in response to our pressing of various buttons correspond to various mathematical calculations that we are able to undertake. Because of the correspondences that we have established, we can interpret the visible outcome as the correct result of a mathematical calculation. But in actual fact, there was no calculation or intellectual process going on at all except for our interpretation of the final result. We were not calculating; the machine was doing all the work. It was not calculating; it was just going through a sequence of intrinsically meaningless physical processes. There was something analogous to calculating going on in the sense that the designers arranged it so that the sequence of physical states of the machine correspond to various stages of a mathematical calculation. But the analogy consists just of the correspondence, no more and no less.

What goes on in the various perceptual systems is, I submit, another example of blind causation. Although these systems are not literally the outcome of intelligent design, they are the outcome of natural selection and thus have acquired the biological function of conveying useful information to the organism. Although the physical causal sequences that result in a sensation are instances of blind causation that contains no intrinsic content at all, they function in such a way that the sensations they produce so depend upon certain facts in the organism's environment that their occurrence is capable of being interpreted by the organism as indicating those facts. The production of a sensation is analogous then to the production of a numeral on the screen of a calculator. Both are the outcomes of blind causation. Both are 'designed' so as to have a certain function based upon correspondences established by the 'designing' process. And both can be interpreted by the intelligent agents who become conscious of them as signifying some fact. There is no more need to suppose that the sensation possess any intrinsic propositional content than to suppose that the numeral on the calculator's screen intrinsically means a number. When we speak of the visual system and the calculator as representing information or as producing outcomes that have propositional content, we are implicitly alluding to the fact that the events that they produce are interpretable by intelligent creatures who possess sufficient background information to impose meaning upon them in view of the physical dependencies in which they are immersed.

NOTES

1. D.M. Armstrong, *Perception and the Physical World* (London: Routledge and Kegan Paul, 1961), p. 114. I recommend this book for a powerful defense of this view.

2. For an excellent discussion of the place of inference in perception see Brand Blanshard, *The Nature of Thought* (London: George Allen and Unwin, 1948), Volume I, Chapter 2.

3. These passages occur at the end of the second meditation. The translation is by Donald Cress of his edition of Descartes' *Meditations on First Philosophy* (Indianapolis, Indiana: Hackett Publishing Co., 1979), pp. 22, 23.

4. For another version of this argument see my *Color and Consciousness: An Essay in Metaphysics* (Philadelphia: Temple University Press, 1989), pp. 71-77.

5. John Locke, *An Essay Concerning Human Understanding*, Bk. II, Ch. xix, par. 1.
6. P.A. Boghossian and J.D. Velleman, "Colour as a Secondary Quality," *Mind*, Vol. XCVIII, Jan. 1989, p. 82n. For claims about the intentionality of sensation, also see Christopher Peacocke, *Sense and Content* (Oxford: Clarendon Press, 1983), pp. 5-9; G.E.M. Anscombe, "The Intentionality of Sensation: A Grammatical Feature," in R.J. Butler (ed.), *Analytical Philosophy, Second Series* (Oxford: Basil Blackwell, 1965); John Searle, *Intentionality, An Essay in the Philosophy of Mind* (Cambridge: Cambridge University Press, 1983), Chapter II.
7. Fred Dretske denies that the fact that smoke is a sign of fire or that smoke indicates fire presupposes interpreters who take smoke to mean fire. He thinks that one thing can indicate something else even though there is no one to whom it indicates. (*Explaining Behavior: Reasons in a World of Causes* (Cambridge, Mass.: The MIT Press, 1988), p. 55). This is quite implausible because causal dependencies exist throughout the universe. Does that mean the meaning exists throughout the universe in the absence of interpreters? A bit later, he formulates his claim so that it is compatible with the indispensability of interpreters. "There is something *in* nature (not merely in the minds that struggle to comprehend nature), some objective, observer-independent fact or set of facts, that forms the basis of one thing's meaning or indicating something about another." (p. 58) I agree that there is an independent basis for natural signification, namely the causal relation between the sign and the signified. But that relation is just *a* condition for signification; it is not sufficient unto itself.
8. The emphasis on intrinsic intentionality is quite explicit in Searle, *op. cit.*, Introduction.
9. For this view see Jerry Fodor, *The Language of Thought* (New York: Thomas Y. Crowell Company, 1975), pp. 44-51; Richard L. Gregory, "Perceptions as Hypotheses," in S.C. Brown (ed.), *Philosophy of Psychology* (New York: Harper and Row, 1974); Gary Hatfield, "Representation and Content in some (Actual) Theories of Perception," *Studies in the History and Philosophy of Science*, Vol. 19, 1988; and Irwin Rock, *The Logic of Perception* (Cambridge, Mass.: The MIT Press, 1983), chapters one and two.
10. William James, *The Principles of Psychology* (Dover Publications, 1950), Volume I, pp. 284-285.
11. Ludwig Wittgenstein, *Philosophical Investigations* (New York: The Macmillan company, 1953), Part II, section xi.
12. Gregory, *op. cit.*, p. 203.
13. *Ibid.*, 209.
14. G. E. M. Anscombe, "Comments on Professor Gregory's Paper" in S.C. Brown, *op. cit.*, pp. 213, 218.
15. Gregory, *op. cit.*, p. 233.
16. *Ibid.*, p. 234; see also Rock, *op. cit.*, pp. 19-20, 32.

CHAPTER 4

A REPRESENTATIVE THEORY OF SENSATION

TOUCH AND TEMPERATURE

I have argued that once we bring the scientific story into the picture, it is implausible to continue to insist on the principle of direct acquaintance implicit in our common sense understanding of seeing. A representational account of perception seems more plausible once we adopt the view that the coming into being of visual perception is a highly mediated causal process, the end result of which is a visual sensation. but there are difficulties in the way of a representative account. One of them emerges as a result of the argument that there is no reason to suppose that sensations embody propositional content. If they do not possess this sort of intrinsic intentionality, how do they come to represent the external world? The second difficulty is founded upon the phenomenon of transparency that Moore emphasized. Visual perception, it appears, goes straight way to its object without any intervening sensation at all. If visual sensations are just a part of a myth of the given, if we have direct access to the external world, then the representative account has no point.

I shall now turn to these issues and try to defend a representational theory of perception. When philosophers and psychologists discuss perception in general, in most cases what they are really discussing is visual perception.[1] Most of the examples employed to illustrate and argue for various theories are visual. It seems to me that the initial implausibility to common sense of the representational theory comes from overemphasizing the visual case. So I shall begin here instead by discussing the perception of heat by the sense of touch. A representational account of the perception of heat is intrinsically plausible even within our common sense view of perception. As we shall see, we need to bring the scientific story into the picture even here, but not for the purpose of establishing a representational account.

Suppose I touch a hot stove and feel its heat. My perception consists of feeling the heat of the stove. In feeling the hot stove and its heat, I learn that the stove is hot. This is a belief based upon the perception but distinguishable from it. I shall consider now the perception itself and put aside the subsequent cognitive achievements based upon it.

If the fingers with which I touched the stove had been anaesthetized, I would have been unable to feel its heat. Mere contact with the stove is insufficient to generate the perception. A necessary condition for feeling something's heat is that one have certain sensations in a part of one's body in contact with it or in contact with the heat radiating from it. Thus in perceiving the stove's heat by touch, I am sensing it, that is I am having a sensation of heat in a part of my body, and, moreover, it is a sensation of that very heat which is in the stove.

What makes this sensation one of heat in general and of this very heat in particular? Whence comes this content? I do not think it profitable to introduce intrinsic intentionality at this point. A much simpler account with fewer mysteries is available. What makes this sensation one of heat is that it is caused or produced by heat; what makes it one of this very heat in the stove is that it is caused by this very heat in the stove. In general, that a type of sensation is of heat just means that it is usually caused by heat. If that type of sensation had, instead, been caused by cold, it would have been a sensation of cold. Thus the representational character of the sensation is founded upon the general dependency relation between it and its typical causes. In that way the sensation comes to function as a sign of heat and to carry the information that the thing felt is hot.

Because of this general causal relation and my subsequent learning about it, I can discover that the stove is hot just by touching it. The sensation I feel triggers the belief that the stove it hot. The belief is based upon the sensation together with the knowledge gained by sight that what I am touching is a stove. The sensation functions as a representation for me of the heat of the stove. The explanation of how it functions as a representation does not require us to bring into play the concept of intrinsic intentionality at all. It possesses no intrinsic propositional content and need not be presumed to do so in order to explain how it delivers to me the information that the stove is hot.

But how do we come to learn that this type of sensation of one of heat? Here is a likely scenario. A child touches a hot stove and receives an unpleasant sensation. Its mother warns it not to touch the stove again because it is hot. Repetitions of similar conversations accustom the child to apply the term "hot" or its equivalent to things from which it receives this type of sensation. It acquires knowledge of the dependency relation between the sensation and things that are hot. It also learns that hot things have heat in them that is capable of radiating out and being felt at a distance. Sooner or later the child, having been guided by the conversations of others, learns to apply heat concepts on its own, now being guided by its own sensations. These sensations now come to mean heat. They come to be the basis on which heat concepts are applied. They acquire a cognitive function; they become the child's foundation for applying heat concepts on its own.

There is not much room for skepticism here. We can understand how the child becomes capable of inferring the existence of something hot on the basis of its sensation. It is true that the belief that there is something hot there is usually triggered by the sensation; it seldom arises as a result of a self-conscious, controlled, self-critical intellectual process. But it deserves to be called an inference because there is a passage of the mind from the sensation together with acquired background knowledge to the belief, a passage of mind that can be evaluated as sound or unsound, valid or invalid, as producing truth or falsehood. It is an inference because our epistemic evaluations apply to it. It is an inference because it is correctable in subsequent instances.

We can also see that Moore's transparency thesis is inapplicable to the perception of heat by touch. Our consciousness does not go straightway to the heat perceived but is mediated by the sensation. The mediating role of the sensation is discernible through introspection.

HEAT

We see, then, that through these early conversations, a child acquires a certain concept of heat and becomes able to identify hot objects on his own via his sensations. The concept of heat that the child possess at this stage is of something that causes sensations of this sort. Sooner or later, the child learns as a result of further conversations together with his own observations that heat is capable of producing other effects such as cooking food, melting candles, and so forth. As the child's knowledge of the powers of heat develop, its concept of heat develops additional content.

But however much content it incorporates, it remains at this stage a concept of a power. Perhaps this accounts for Locke's view of secondary qualities according to which heat, along with color, sound, taste, and smell are mere powers of bodies to produce certain effects, the most salient of which are the sensations in the minds of perceivers. Locke recognized that the secondary qualities which he identified with certain of the causal powers of bodies are founded upon the underlying microstructures of bodies; he thought that these microstructures consisted of minute bodies or corpuscles that possessed primary qualities only; today we would think that the heat of a body is founded upon the motion of its constituent molecules.[2]

It is one thing to say that a hot body possess certain causal powers, and quite another to claim that heat is nothing but such powers. The former is true; the latter is founded upon a mistake. Locke assumed that the concept that one has of something determines what that thing is; in his terms the concept incorporates a nominal essence. So the child, by virtue of possessing a concept of heat knows the nominal essence of heat. Locke distinguished the nominal from the real essence; the nominal belongs to our concept, and the real essence is the hidden corpuscular structure of bodies that explains their observable characteristics.[3] But since Locke thought that heat is just a quality, not a substance, there is no distinction to be drawn between its nominal and real essence. All the secondary qualities are nothing but causal powers.

Locke's view embodies two errors. The first is to suppose that the concept of an item that a person possesses invariably incorporates information about its nature. Locke was writing at a time when what he called the corpuscularian hypothesis was becoming entrenched in the explanatory system of science. This hypothesis enabled scientists to distinguish between the observable features of bodies and the underlying structures that performed most of the explanatory work. The nature of a thing is determined by what does most of the explanatory work. Thus the observable features by and large could no longer be thought of as determining a thing's nature. This fact is prefigured in Locke's distinctions between real and nominal essence and primary and secondary qualities. But he did not take the final step of recognizing that the concept of an item whose content includes just those observable features that help us identify it and ascertain its presence is not necessarily a concept that contains information about its nature. The concept need not be a concept of essence in any sense. If we distinguish between a recognitional concept that contains enough information to identify an item and an essential concept that informs us of its nature according to the explanatory framework entrenched at the time, then Locke's initial error was to mistake a recognitional concept of heat for an essential concept. The child's concept is recognitional, and thus one cannot determine what heat is by analysing it.

Locke's second error is to think of heat as a quality of bodies, if by a quality we think of a category in contrast to the categories of substance, process, event, stuff and so forth. It is true that the word "hot" is an adjective and thus linguistically may be thought of as standing for a quality. But what makes something hot is the heat in it, and, from a common sense point of view, heat is something that can radiate through space, that can be transferred from one body to another, that can produce changes in objects, etc. We tend to think of heat as a stuff which unlike other stuffs such as water or gold, is naturally in process. The common sense category that best fits our pre-scientific understanding of heat is that of process-stuff. This is rather vague, but our common sense understanding of the nature of heat is not very precise to begin with. Once we bring science into play and realise that heat is a form of molecular motion, our common sense categorization is superseded. This is a nice example of how the shift from common sense to a scientific scheme not only deepens our conception of something's nature but also produces a change in the applicable categories. In fact we have two categoreal shifts from respect to heat. The first is the transition from the child's (and Locke's) conception of heat as a causal power to the more developed conception of heat as an actual entity that does work, a process-stuff; the second is the shift from the category of process-stuff to the scientific categories of molecular motion and energy.

In any case, Thomas Reid had a finer appreciation of the status of heat in our conceptual scheme than did Locke. Here is an example of what he has to say on the issue:

> The qualities in bodies which we call *heat* and *cold* are unknown. They are only conceived by us, as unknown causes or occasions of the sensations to which we give the same names. But, though common sense says nothing of the nature of these qualities, it plainly dictates the existence of them....It is the business of philosophers to investigate, by

> proper experiments and induction, what heat and cold are in bodies...; for common sense says nothing on the one side or the other. But, whatever be the nature of that quality in bodies which we call *heat*, we certainly know this, that it cannot in the least resemble the sensation of heat.[4]

Reid recognized that our common sense conceptual scheme leaves us ignorant of the nature of heat and that it is the job of science (which he calls "philosophy") to tell us what heat really is. From the common sense standpoint, heat is a something I know not what which is capable of causing certain characteristic sensations. We know some of its relational-causal properties, but have no reliable information about its intrinsic nature.

When Reid says that heat in itself does not resemble our sensation of heat and thus implies that we should distinguish heat from the sensations it produces, he probably had Berkeley's theory of heat in mind. In his *Three Dialogues between Hylas and Philonous*, Berkeley has Philonous assert: "But is not the most vehement and intense degree of heat a very great pain?" In the interest of defending his immaterialist philosophy, Berkeley here tries to blur the distinction between the objective features of bodies and the subjective sensings of them.

At first, Hylas insists on the distinction that Berkeley want to blur: "Hold, Philonous, I fear I was out in yielding intense heat to be a pain. it should seem rather, that pain is something distinct from heat and the consequence or effect of it." But Philonous responds: "Is not the heat immediately perceived?....And the pain?....Seeing that they are both immediately perceived at the same time, and the fire affects you only with one simple, or uncompounded idea, it follows that this same simple idea is both the intense heat immediately perceived, and the pain; and consequently, that the intense heat immediately perceived, is nothing distinct from a particular sort of pain."[5]

In this response, the issue about the nature of heat shifts to the question of immediate perception. For Berkeley, heat is a sensible thing, that is, it is something that can be perceived or, more specifically, felt. Philonous had earlier asserted:

> By *sensible things* I mean those only which are perceived by sense, and...in truth the senses perceive nothing which they do not perceive

> immediately: for they make no inferences. The deducing therefore of causes or occasions from effects and appearances, which alone are perceived by sense, entirely relates to reason.[6]

The contrast that Berkeley intends between immediate and mediate perception is between the non-inferential awareness of a quality and the awareness of something that is suggested or signified by what we immediately perceive. Because, in feeling the heat of an object, I do not thereby infer its presence, the heat is immediately perceived and the way is open, Berkeley thinks, to identify heat with the sensation of heat. For isn't the sensation the only item that is immediately perceived?

The major error in Berkeley's account lies in his conflating mediation with inference. As we saw in the previous section, the perception of heat is highly mediated. Not only is there a complex causal process including events in the nervous system that underlies heat perception, but a sensation of heat is indispensable. But it doesn't follow that in feeling the heat, one thereby infers its presence from the sensation. Such an inference may be involved in arriving at the judgment that something is hot, but the judgment should not, as we saw, be confused with the perception that triggers it. It is sufficient for the perception that the heat in the object causes the sensation. Since one's perceptual consciousness of the heat is mediated by the sensation, it is perfectly reasonable to say that one is directly consciousness of the sensation and only indirectly conscious of the heat. But this contrast between direct and indirect consciousness should not be confused with the contrast between perception and inference.

A final question. When someone judges that something is hot on the basis of his feeling a hot object, is it correct to say that he *knows* that the object is hot? Does touch perception constitute a ground of knowledge? Cartesian doubts are possible here. It is logically possible that the sensation of heat is non-veridical; one can have the sensation without the object one is touching being hot at all. The inference from the sensation to the heat is not certain or conclusive. So if one were in the situation of trying to determine whether or not one knows that the object is hot or even that there is any object there at all that could be hot just on the basis of the sensation, one would have to conclude that one could not be sure, and that therefore one does not possess knowledge.

These skeptical doubts, however, confuse two different issues. One issue is whether the belief based upon the perception of heat counts as knowledge. It seems to me that it does. Since the hot object is actually perceived, then the sensation of heat is actually caused by the object, so the belief is true, and it is acquired in a way which is not accidental and is generated in virtue of contact with the very fact that makes it true. It is hard to see what else is required for knowledge in this case. The other issue is whether or not one can tell that one has knowledge if the only information one has available is that provided by the sensation. Under those constraints, I think that one can say that one does not know that one knows that there is a hot object that one is touching. Thus the belief that one's belief is a case of knowledge may not itself be a case of knowledge; but that does not prevent the initial belief from being a case of knowledge.

TASTE AND SMELL

Olfactory and gustatory perception bear certain similarities to the perception of heat. We think, for example, of the taste of a tomato as some 'feature' it possesses that is usually manifested in the mouth and on the tongue. A claim to the effect that this sensation is the sensation of the taste of this tomato implies that it is caused by whatever it is in the tomato that constitutes its taste. What there is in the tomato, its taste, that is responsible for producing the sensation is generally unknown to us unless we happen to have knowledge of the tomato's chemical makeup. In its absence, all we know of the taste is the sensation it produces. The same point applies to smell. The sensation of smell is generated by sniffing the air in proximity to the object. Smell sensations are vaguely located in the area of the nose and cannot be located with the precision of taste sensations. The smell of an object consists in an aspect of its chemical makeup, but this is unknown to us in the absence of scientific investigation.

There is an interesting difference between taste and smell. An object's taste is a 'feature' that it possesses within it; the object can produce its sensations of taste only when it is placed in contact with the inside of the mouth and the tongue. But an object's smell is not confined to the object; it is also something that the object 'gives off' so that contact with it is not necessary to obtain the sensation.

There is an interesting difference between taste and smell on the one hand and heat on the other. Even prior to our scientific knowledge, heat reveals its presence in a variety of distinct effects upon surrounding objects and not only in sensory effects. But for the most part smell and taste reveal themselves only through their sensory effects. Since smells and tastes are chemically constituted, they are capable of producing effects other than the sensory, but these are not much noted by us.

Moore's transparency thesis is no more applicable to smell and taste than it is to the perception of heat. Our consciousness with respect to all three does not go straightway to an objective feature of material things but is mediated by a sensation. Because, in each case, the sensation is generally dependent for its generation upon an external cause, it is true to say that the sensation is a sign of its cause and represents it to us. Therefore, for these senses, a representative theory of perception is correct.

We can also see that, for these senses at least, Descartes was mistaken in assimilating sensation to thought. What makes a certain sensation one of heat is that it is caused by heat. The intentionality or representative function of the sensation is not intrinsic but is a consequence of its external causal relations. However, the thought of the heat of an object is not directly causally dependent upon its heat. For example, I may be led to think of the heat of the sun by reading a book on astronomy. Unlike our sensations, our thoughts are relatively independent of the causal activity of the objects they represent. Thus our thoughts of objects, whatever they are, should not be classified as signs. They may very well possess intrinsic intentionality. But a representative theory of perception, as developed here, is a theory of signs, not a theory of intrinsic intentionality.

Thomas Reid point out that we have a tendency to confuse the features of our sensations with the features of the objects that cause them. I think that there is something to his claim. Unless I am thinking of objects in terms of the scientific theories about them, when I think of the heat of an object, I find myself usually thinking of features of the sensation. Similarly for smell and taste. There is a psychological tendency to objectify sensory qualities and to think of them as qualities of their causes. But, as Reid pointed out, this is a mistake. There is no significant resemblance between the sensory qualities and those motions or chemicals in the material things that cause them. Perhaps these objectifying tendencies are important in explaining how it is that perceptual consciousness is a consciousness of an external world.

One historically popular version of the representative theory of perception brings sense data into the picture. For purposes of this discussion, by a sense datum I shall mean a mental particular which possesses various qualities; the qualities that it actually possesses are those that the material object perceived seems to possess. Thus when an object looks blue, according to the sense datum account, there is a sense datum that actually is blue and of which the perceiver is conscious. Although the account offered here of the perception of heat, tastes, and smells resembles a sense datum account, it has a significant dissimilarity that disqualifies it from being one. The similarity is that according to both accounts, in perceiving the heat or the smell or the taste of an object, there is indeed a mental particular of which the perceiver is directly conscious. However, unlike the sense datum account, on my account there is no reason to suppose that the sensation possesses any of those features that it leads us to think the object has. When an object feels hot, for example, there is no reason to suppose that the sensation of heat literally is hot. Thus the sensation of heat is not a sense datum. To mark the difference from sense datum theories, I shall label the view here espoused *the representative theory of sensation* (RTS).

According to RTS, sensations have features that we are capable of being conscious of and of directly discriminating from other features. This aspect of the theory has a certain consequence for the mind-body problem. Let "s" be the name of a particular sensation of smell and "F" the name of its directly discriminable feature or features. Thus it is true that s is F, and the person having the sensation s can directly verify that it is true. Now consider the claim of the mind-brain identity theory that sensations are brain processes. On this view, s is identical with some brain process b. Thus s and b must have all their properties in common; therefore b is F. Yet F is not a property that would be classified as one of the physical or neural features of b. If what goes on in the brain causes what happens in our sensory life, then something going on in the brain causes something to exemplify F. But this causal claim does not show that it is a brain process that exemplifies F. So either there are sensory events that are not brain processes and that have there own discriminable properties, or there are sensory events that are brain processes that have special non-physical properties. Either there is no b that is identical to s, or, if there is a b that is identical to s, its properties include both physical and mental features. In any case, a radical reduction of the mental to the physical is blocked.

SOUNDS

Consider sounds that the violinist makes in a concert hall. They are not features of the violin or the violinist but something that she produces by rubbing the bow against the strings. We think of the sounds as radiating from their source where the violinist stands and filling the hall. Sounds in the common sense picture are process-stuffs, more like heat than like qualities of objects as we take colors and shapes to be. If I sit near the violinist, the sounds she produces appear quite loud, but, from the rear of the hall, I may barely be able to hear them at all. The very same sound, we think, can appear loud to a greater or less degree.

But this common sense picture does not survive once we bring the scientific account into play. What the violinist actually produces when she rubs the bow against the strings are vibrations in the strings that cause air waves that travel throughout the hall. These waves cause changes in our ears, auditory nerves, and brain, the result of which is that we hear sounds. By analogy with the other senses that have already been discussed, the sound we are directly conscious of in hearing the violinist play is a sensation, a sensory effect that exists only when we are affected. It itself does not fill the hall but possesses only a mental and subjective reality. Our imputation of objective status to it is an error that we cannot help making. The pressure waves are objective; they fill the hall; but they are not the sounds we hear; rather they are among the causal conditions for the production of those sensations that are the sounds we hear. This is another example of how the scientific story tends to undermine the common sense of the matter.

What are the objects of hearing? What do we hear in the concert hall? We hear the violinist; we hear her playing the violin; and we hear the sounds she makes by playing the violin. The objects of hearing consist of the source of the sound, the event of the source's producing the sound, and the sound that is produced. The common sense view of the matter is that all three belong to the 'external' world; we are aware of the sounds and, through them, of the source and originating events. The scientific story undermines the common sense account by providing reasons for supposing that sound itself belongs to the subjective side of the situation, that it exists in consciousness alone and is directly caused by those brain events that are themselves caused by the impact of the pressure waves upon the auditory system.

A view that fits in better with the common sense of the matter is that the auditory system causes our awareness or consciousness of sound, but not the sounds themselves. The sounds belong to the objective side; it is only the consciousness of them that is subjective. There are two alternatives here: (1) According to the first, the sound itself is said to be identical to the pressure waves caused by the source. (2) On the second, the sound is something over and above the pressure waves to which it is correlated. But neither alternative is plausible. The first fails because the directly discriminable features of sounds such as pitch and timbre, although correlated to a significant degree with certain features of the waves, can hardly be said to *be* those features. For example, the greater the frequency of the waves, the higher the pitch of the sound that is heard. Yet there is no resemblance between the pitch and the number of cycles per unit of time. The second is implausible because there is no reasonable way to determine how and why the sounds came into existence in addition to the waves. Do the waves cause the sounds? How? By what mechanism? And if by some miracle they cause the sounds, the waves do all the work in explaining how hearing occurs; the sounds drop out of the picture.

Once the scientific story is available, the common sense picture loses all plausibility. The auditory system resembles a frequency analyser, and there are broad correlations between sound qualities and the impulses that the inner ear produces in the brain. Thus the effects in consciousness should have the diversity that sounds actually have rather than the sameness that consciousness is supposed to have according to the transparency thesis. So the supposition that the subjective side of hearing consists of 'mere' consciousness of objective sounds cannot reasonably be made to square with our best accounts of how hearing is caused.

When we hear sounds our common sense beliefs are mistaken in the following ways: first we think, incorrectly, that the sounds we hear are objective process-stuffs. Second, we think that the sound that each of us hears is numerically the same even though it can sound differently at different distances from the source. But in fact, what each of us is directly conscious of are distinct mental particulars produced by our own personal auditory mechanisms. The differences in appearances are really different features of these private particulars that we can directly discriminate.

With respect to hearing, RTS and the sense datum theory coincide. According to RTS, sounds are sensations with introspectible qualities. According to the sense datum approach, sounds are sense data with directly apprehensible qualities. Both claim that sounds are mental particulars with qualities of which we are directly conscious. The reason why they coincide here although they have elsewhere been found to diverge is due to the fact that the properties which sounds appear to possess via the sensations of them are properties which the sensations do in fact possess. In the case of heat, for example, although the sensation was of heat, it was not itself hot. There is, in the case of heat, smell, and taste, a divergence between the objective property that the sensation signifies and the discriminable features of the sensation itself. But in the case of sound, once we recognize that we are mistaken in supposing that the properties of sounds are properties of an objective stuff, the divergence disappears. The sensation of a certain tone exemplifies that very tone.

NOTES

1. Thomas Reid is a distinguished exception. In his *An Inquiry into the Human Mind* (in the first volume of his *Philosophical Works*, ed. Sir William Hamilton), the chapter immediately following the introduction is on smelling. Then follow chapters and tasting, hearing, and touch, and only after these does he discuss seeing.
2. For Locke's distinction between primary and secondary qualities see his *An Essay Concerning Human Understanding*, Book II, chapter viii. See also the discussion of Locke's view in my *Color and Consciousness, An Essay in Metaphysics* (Philadelphia: Temple University Press, 1989), chapters ii and iii.
3. For Locke's discussion of nominal and real essences, see his *Essay*, Book III, chapter iii.
4. Thomas Reid, *An Inquiry into the Human Mind* in his *Philosophical Works*, ed. Sir William Hamilton, Volume I, p. 119.
5. George Berkeley, *Three Dialogues between Hylas and Philonous* (Indianapolis: Hackett Publishing Co., 1984), p. 12.
6. *Ibid.*, p. 11.

CHAPTER 5

COLOR SUBJECTIVELY CONSIDERED

VISION AND COLOR

Vision resembles hearing in this way: mere reflection upon the experience fails to show that the objects were are directly conscious of in the experience are bodily sensations or even that they are sensations to be ascribed to the subject at all. We required an argument to show that the sound of the violinist is a sensory effect and not an occupant of the concert hall. The argument depended upon premises drawn from the science of sound which are unavailable to mere reflective common sense. If, as the materialist claims, sensations of sound are brain processes and thus have a definite bodily location, this fact too is unavailable to reflective common sense and depends upon scientific consideration at least.

When I look at, for example, a red tomato, among the features that I am directly conscious of are, as far as reflective common sense is concerned, *its* color and shape. The specific features accessible to vision are color, shape, size, motion and various spatial (and perhaps temporal) relations among the objects located in the visual field. These are features of and relations among bodies, or so it seems. The color that we see when we look at the tomato ostensibly belongs to the tomato and is as objective as its shape. Whereas mere reflection upon experience reveals that our perceptual awareness of heat is mediated by a bodily sensation, reflection fails to discover any mediation as far as visual perception is concerned. Our concept of color is, accordingly, a concept of a feature of bodies, of something predicated of bodies that they exemplify independently of being perceived. We do not think, for example, that when we cease to look at the tomato, it loses its color.

Locke seems to deny these deliverances of simple reflection:

> Let us consider the red and white colours in *Porphyre*: Hinder light but from striking on it, and its Colours Vanish; it no longer produces any such *Ideas* in us: Upon the return of Light, it produces these

> appearances on us again. Can any one think any real alterations are made in the *Porphyre*, by the presence or absence of Light; and that those *Ideas* of whiteness and redness, are really in *Porphyre* in the light, when 'tis plain *it has no colour in the dark*?[1]

But it is clear that what Locke means when he says that objects lose their colors in the dark is that they no longer appear or look colored. Of course, the appearances of color vanish when visual perception ceases; but it does not follow from that fact alone that color ceases. To be fair to Locke, this passage appears at a point in the chapter after he presented arguments intended to show that visible color resides in the appearances. So he may very well have a right to such a conclusion. But we have not approached that stage in the argument as yet; what we are concerned to present here is our common understanding of color, not the understanding that may emerge subsequent to scientific and philosophical arguments.

Color has certain aspects that tend to show that it is a quality of bodies and other aspects that tend to show that it is a stuff. It is a quality in so far as it is predicated of bodies; moreover we do not think of an object's color as being among the items it is composed of. A pink ice cube (to use Wilfrid Sellars' example[2]) is pink through and through but it is composed of solidified water molecules and enough red paint to make it look pink. But colors also seem to possess stuff-like aspects. For example, the color of the tomato *covers* its entire outer surface and, indeed, *permeates* it through and through. When you are tinting the water in order to produce a colored ice cube, you may put more red in the mixture in order to make it appear in the desired way. Of course, one puts more red in the mixture by putting more red paint in it, but the addition of red paint is a means of adding more red. The blue sky is not only blue, its blue color *fills* it through and through; every visible part has blue in it. The color *extends* throughout the visible sky and is essentially and necessarily extensive in nature. In our concept of color, extensiveness and relation to space are necessary and not merely accidental features.

VISUAL SENSATIONS

Given our concept of color as an objective feature of bodies together with the ostensibly unmediated nature of visual perception, it would seem that visual perception is the one case in which Moore's transparency thesis obtains. Yet I do not think that it is true even in this case. There are sufficient analogies between the visual and the other perception modalities to cast doubt upon the naive realism implicit in our common sense assumptions.

In our consciousness of heat, for example, we can distinguish between our perceptual awareness of the heat we feel and the sensation of heat that mediates the perceptual awareness. There is a distinction here between perceptual and sensory consciousness, between the perception of a feature of an object and the sensation that contact with the object produces. A similar distinction can be drawn in the visual case. It is not founded as it is in the case of heat upon our awareness of a bodily sensation inextricably involved in the perception. In seeing something, we are not aware of any sensations located in or near our eyes. However, within the common sense framework, we come to understand that there can be and frequently are variations in the ways in which the colors and shapes of objects appear even though their actual colors and shapes remain the same. An orange object placed in red light may look red; a straight stick placed in water may look bent. Put on a pair of blue tinted glasses and, for a time, everything you see looks blue. The appearance of visual objects is a function not just of their objective features but also of the surroundings, the ambient light, the position and orientation of the observer, and the condition of his sense organs and visual system generally. We learn, even without the benefit of scientific understanding, that enormous variations in the ways things look is compatible with relative stability in their objective character. Our concept of a material think is a concept of a type of item that can be apprehended from different and distinct points of view. One would thus expect a multiplicity of appearances corresponding to the multiplicity of point of view.[3]

However, the correspondence is not exact. The gestalt psychologists have emphasized that changes in appearance do not occur as frequently as do changes in local visual stimulation. There are various visual constancies—in color, in brightness, in size and shape. For example, a white object placed in a shadow may still look white. A tall man receding into the distance still appears tall. They have also claimed that these constancies are not determined solely by our judgments but belong to sensory consciousness. It is not the case that the white paper's continuing to appear white in the shadow consists just in our persistent belief that it is white. We may have such a belief based upon our having learned that objects do not change colors just because the illumination has changed. But sensory consciousness is not just a matter of belief. There are basic constancies in the sensations themselves that are not a product of prior learning.[4]

According to a more recent study, there is an experimental and theoretical basis for the claim that apparent or perceived colors "do not depend slavishly on the light from each object, sensed independently of all the other things in the world, but on a comparison of the light from an object and its surroundings."[5] Color constancy has a certain biological value that suggests the possibility that it is a product of natural selection. Organisms use colors to identify objects with respect to their potential benefits and harms, e.g. as nourishing food, as hostile predators, and so forth. "Yet unreliable distinctions are useless. Indeed they are a hindrance. They are busyness without meaning and so are equivalent to noise. This gives value to color constancy. The ability to recognize things would be lessened if their color changed simply because of a change in illumination."[6]

Yet the existence of the constancies does not affect the basic point that there occur significant deviations between how things appear and how they really are. There are well known optical illusions; there are hallucinations. The constancies hold only up to a point. And they can be overcome by isolating the perceived object from its surroundings to prevent our visual system from making comparisons. And if we change the local stimulation sufficiently as in the case of the stick that looks bent in water and in other cases too numerous to mention, a multitude of failures of veridicality can be generated.

Even when no failure of veridicality is in question, we can distinguish the look of a thing as a fact that is logically and conceptually independent of its real properties. That this looks blue does not entail that it is blue; that it is blue does not entail that it looks blue. How a thing looks is a fact dependent upon the observer. Without beings capable of being sensitively affected, there would be no way that things look, no visual appearances.

Yet there are those who have argued that the familiar facts pointed out in this section do not justify taking the subjective turn in the case of vision. The fact that the existence of, say, the appearance of the bent stick depends upon the observer in part does not imply that the look of the thing has subjective status; in fact it does not imply that there is nothing bent that is being seen. If we stick to the deliverances of immediate experience, there is something bent that is being seen, and there is nothing subjective about that. Even a camera will record a bent stick. Consider this passage from Dewey:

> Suppose we take...an out and out illusion, say of Zollner's lines. These are experienced as convergent; they are 'truly' parallel. If things are what they are experienced as being, how can the distinction be drawn between illusion and the true state of the case? There is no answer to this question except by sticking to the fact that the experience of the lines as divergent is a concrete qualitative thing or *that*....The lines of *that* experience *are* divergent; not merely *seem* so.[7]

In another place, Dewey claims that he accepts "a thorough going naive realism."[8] On the basis of his comments on Zollner's lines, a thorough going naive realism implies that when something looks to be such and such, then there really is something, a quale or sense datum, that *is* such and such. That is what makes the realism naive. And what makes it a form of realism is the denial of a subjective or mental status to the experience.

In our earlier discussion of the perception of sound, we saw that once the scientific story is added to explain the causes of auditory perception, it becomes implausible to suppose that the sounds we hear possess the objective status attributed to them by common sense. But the same point applies to the appearance of a bent stock. A mind-independent bent-stick sense datum has no explanatory role to play; it drops out of the picture in favor of an inner sensory effect. Dewey says that "pragmatism is content to take its stand with science."[9] But science taken literally moves us away from naive realism. Nor is it open to Dewey to attribute absolute epistemological priority to the deliverances of immediate experience. For he is a pragmatist and hence a fallibilist and thus is not permitted to attribute the degree of certainty to judgments of immediate experience that they would be required to have to outweigh the scientific considerations against naive realism. For a fallibilist, no belief can be held come what may.

VISUAL SENSING AND VISUAL SENSE DATA

These considerations lend plausibility to the supposition that in vision as well as in the other senses, there is a distinction to be drawn between perceptual and sensory consciousness. It is a reasonable hypothesis, then, that the occurrence of visual sensations is a necessary condition of having something in sight. I do not want to imply that these sensations are themselves the real or genuine objects of sight; that would be a mistake; what we see are just the things we normally take ourselves to be seeing: tables and books and people and trees and meadows and dogs and cats. The distinction between perceptual and sensory consciousness simply means that the occurrence of sensations is one of the intervening or mediating conditions that are necessary for these things to be seen. The considerations raised above tend to undermine our naive principle of direct acquaintance; seeing is the result of a highly mediated process including events within the sense organs and nervous system but also including elements of consciousness, the visual sensations themselves with features we can be acquainted with.

That there is a distinction between perceptual and sensory consciousness, and that the latter is an essential means to and constituent of the former should not be taken to imply that in seeing something we infer the existence of what we see from the visual sensation with which we are acquainted. Sense perception as I have argued is not an intrinsically cognitive affair and should be distinguished from the judgments and beliefs which, in human beings, are its characteristic results and accompaniments. Rather, the object we see is one of the causes of the sensation; its causal role in the series of events that culminate in the sensation contributes to the explanation of how we see it. If the sensation occurs without the object playing a causal role, then we fail to see it even if we think we do.

Should the visual sensation be interpreted as the occurrence of a sense datum? If we take the sense datum route, then we are committed to the claim that the sensation actually possesses those features which the object appears to possess. So if an object looks blue and square, then the associated sense datum is blue and square. But this is manifestly implausible. There is no reason at all to suppose when something looks blue and square there is an item that is blue and square occurring in the brain or in the mind. The view that there are visual sense data whose occurrence is necessary for seeing things leads to insurmountable and intractable problems for almost any theory of the mind. For the materialistic mind-brain identity theory, it leads to the implausible supposition that colored patches occur in the nervous system whenever we have something in sight. For the Cartesian dualist it leads to the contradiction that spatially extended colored particulars can occur 'in' an unextended mental substance. The sense datum interpretation of visual sensation is a dead end.

There is, however, a strand within the sense datum tradition represented in some of the works of such thinkers as Berkeley, Russell, and Dewey that denies that sense data are literally located in the mind. For Berkeley, the only way in which sense data are in the mind is that they are presented to the mind. Whereas Berkeley thought, however, that the existence of sense data depends upon their being perceived, Russell, in some of his early writings, accepted that there could be unsensed sense data. For both Berkeley and Russell, the sense datum hypothesis was an indispensable component of their phenomenalistic projects of reducing physical objects to phenomenal objects. However, the varied ingenious attempts carried out in this century to show that groupings of phenomenal objects, sense data of various sorts, can do the job of the objects of common sense and science so that the latter can be interpreted as logical constructions out of the former, have not proved themselves successful. Phenomenalistic projects are no longer much discussed; the direction of interest has moved toward realism. We need physical objects for numerous explanatory purposes. But if physical objects are merely permanent possibilities of sensation as Mill characterized them, it is hard to understand how they could satisfactorily play an explanatory role. How could a mere possibility possess any causal efficacy? How could a possible moon explain actual tides? In addition, after the criticisms of Quine and others, it is no longer accepted that the theories of science and the conceptual scheme of every day life can be analysed without remainder in phenomenalistic terms.

Within a realistic framework, as the one adopted in this discussion, there is no need for Russell's or Berkeley's sense data. Physical objects and events do all the explaining of sense perception up to the occurrence of the inner sensation, the point at which the mind-body problem begins. So neither the subjective nor objective versions of the sense datum approach are any longer promising points of departure for an understanding of visual perception or of the foundations of human knowledge.

THE PROBLEM OF VISUAL SENSING

Suppose that I am looking at a certain object that is of a particular shade of blue and it looks blue to me. We can express this situation by saying that the statements formulated by means of these sentences:

(1) This is blue.
(2) This looks blue.

are both true. In (1), an object is described as exemplifying a color of a certain hue. In (2) there is no implication at all that the object or anything else for that matter exemplifies that color. In both sentences, the word "blue" is used with the same meaning; in both a certain hue is designated. Neither sentence differs with respect to what "blue" represents. Because of this semantic identity, it is not plausible to suppose that the meaning of blue in one of the sentences is more fundamental than in the other so that the latter should be analysed in terms of the former. Because, as we suppose, both (1) and (2) are true, then this really does have the very same color that it looks to have. To that extent the visual experience formulated in (2) is veridical. And we can see that perceptual veridicality implies an identity between the character that appears and the character actually exemplified.

Even though there is a semantic identity, we can see that there is a difference between the way a color occurs in the fact represented by (1) and the way it occurs in the fact represented by (2). In the first, it occurs by way of exemplification; in the second it occurs, if at all, in the way of presentation. The semantic identity is consistent with this metaphysical difference. In fact there could not be this difference in the mode of occurrence of the same color if there were not this semantic identity.

The question arises whether it is possible to provide an account of (2) that would clarify its meaning. What does it mean to say that something *looks* in a certain way? One suggestion is that (2) should be analysed as:

(3) This looks the way that things that are blue usually (normally, frequently, characteristically) look.

Because the term "looks" occurs in (3), this suggestion should not be thought of as an analysis of the meaning of "looks" in (2). What (3) accomplishes is that it ties the identity of the character presented to states of affairs in which it is exemplified. What it implies when generalized to apply to any character is that no unexemplified character can be presented. Because the account of color that I shall present in what follows is incompatible with this implication. I shall now show that (3) is not equivalent in meaning to (2).

Consider a possible world in which something is blue if and only if it is spherical. In this universe, things that are blue will normally look both blue and spherical. Now suppose that one of these blue spherical objects is bathed in red light so that it appears purple. In this universe, it is true that:

(4) This looks purple.

Therefore, in this universe, (2) is false. But also suppose that the light has not changed the way the object's shape appears so that:

(5) This looks circular.

Because circular things are blue in this world, then (3) is true even though the object does not look blue. It is possible for (3) to be true and (2) false, so they are not equivalent in meaning.

This example brings out the fact that there is no such thing as the way something looks in general; rather something looks the way it does in some very specific way; in order to characterize the way something looks it is necessary to designate the specific way it looks. It would be better, then, to replace (3) by

(3') This looks the way things that are blue usually look when they look blue.

Unlike (3), (3') designates the specific way the thing is supposed to look. However, (3') fails as an analysis since it makes use of the very concept expressed by "looks blue" that we were trying to explain in the first place.

As an account of (2), both (3) and (3') involve an entirely mistaken approach. What must be true when I utter (2) and succeed in making a true statement is that a certain shade of blue is presented to me when I see an object. I am able to ascertain the truth of (2) because I know what "blue" means and thus I know what color it designates and know what that color looks like and because I am sufficiently attentive to my experience so that the fact that the thing looks blue to me leads me to assert (2). In asserting (2), I do not imply that anything has that color; I do not imply that this thing I am looking at or any other thing for that matter is blue. Moreover, while there may be many true comparisons between how this thing looks and how other things look, it is not the standard job of (2) to make any such comparisons. When I say, for example, that this looks spherical, though there may be many true comparisons that I could make between this and other spherical things, my assertion does not make or imply any such comparisons. Why should "This looks blue" be any different on this score than "This looks spherical"?

How shall we understand the difference between (2) and (4)? They represent, in the first place, numerically different sensations obtained by seeing the same object at different times in different lights. And these sensations are not only numerically different, they are type different as well, that is, they are presentations of different colors, in the one case a shade of blue and in the other a shade of purple. (2) and (4) represent distinct states of affairs. The only difference between them (other than that they occur at different times) is that one involves a presentation of a shade of blue and the other a presentation of a shade of purple. But there is a puzzle here. One might argue that a color or, for that matter, any character, exists only in so far as it is exemplified, that is, only in so far as something actually has it. But neither (2) nor (4) assert or imply that their respective colors are exemplified. There are possible worlds in which both are true even though nothing is blue and nothing is purple. So how can items that do not exist contribute to the differences among states of affairs that do exist? How can items that do not exist even occur in the mode of presentation in existing states of affairs?

THE ADVERBIAL THEORY OF COLOR SENSING

There is an interesting and ingenious theory of sensing sometimes called the adverbial theory that may be used to solve this problem.[10] It says that when a term such as "blue" that is used to designate a sensible feature is used to describe an appearance as in (2), then it should be interpreted not as an adjective representing a feature of bodies but as an adverb designating a certain manner of sensing. On the adverbial interpretation, (2) and (4) should be reformulated as:

(2') I am sensing this bluely.
(4') I am sensing this purplely.

The point of transforming adjectives into adverbs is to communicate that color terms (and sensible feature terms generally), when they occur in appearance statements, designate properties of sensations or events of sensing, not properties that could be possessed by bodies. Thus color terms possess a semantic duality; they mean one thing when ascribed to bodies, another when ascribed to sensations.

The adverbial theory easily resolves the problem of visual sensing. If (2) and (4) are true, it follows, according to the adverbial theory, that color terms designate characters that are exemplified, the items that exemplify them being sensations. So if colors exist only when exemplified, then the states of affairs represented in (2) and (4) are distinguished from one another by reference to constituents that actually exist.

One immediate difficulty with the adverbial theory is implied by what I have already insisted upon, namely that there is no semantic duality in the ordinary use of color terms. The world "blue" means the same in (1) and (2); it designates the same property in both. They differ only with respect to their implications regarding the exemplification of the color. There is no suggestion that "blue" in (2) represents an entity that is categoreally different from that represented in (1). Thus, whatever the virtues of the adverbial theory, it cannot succeed as an account of the meanings of color terms in their standard use in natural language.

It is open to the adverbial theorist to concede this semantic point while denying its significance as a criticism. She may argue as follows: "Even if the theory fails to be correct as an account of the ordinary meanings of color terms, it is, nevertheless, correct as an account of the nature of color sensing. When something looks blue to me, I am having a visual sensation that has an introspectible property that is distinguishable from the property possessed by something's looking purple. Even if the terms "blue" and "purple" do not designate these sensory features as they are ordinarily used, they can be converted to technical terms and stipulated to designate them. The differences in the colors of bodies are parallel to the differences among the sensations we have when we look at them, so it is perfectly appropriate to preempt our color vocabulary to describe the sensations as well."

Suppose that I am looking at something blue, that I see its color, and thus say "That's blue." The color that I am ascribing to the object that I see is the very same as the color that I see; it is the color that I am, ostensibly, directly conscious of. I can attend to the object's color as well as the object. The object not only is blue, it looks blue to me, here and now. That is not only a fact about the object and its color but also a fact about me. When I attend to this fact about me, the color feature that I am attending to is the very same item as the feature that I ascribed to the object when I said "That's blue." When I attended to the object on the one hand and then attended to my sensation on the other, I can find no difference with respect to blue; in both cases, a particular shade of blue is presented. In fact, attending to the object and attending to the sensation do not seem to be cases of attending to different things even though we think of the first as a case of visual perception and the second as a case of introspection. That they are different things in the case of veridical perception is a conclusion one comes to on the basis of argument and is not something that is determined by inspection. What I can tell from inspection, once the distinction between sensation and object is established, is that the color that appears is the very same feature as the one I take to be exemplified by the object that appears.

Thus the adverbial theorist's claim about what is introspectively distinguishable does not seem to be correct. The adverbial theorist has claimed to have discovered by introspection certain features of visual sensation that correspond to colors for which we have no names and has decided to use color terms in a new way to mark this discovery. But there do not seem to be the right things in the sensation to discover. Perhaps this explains why color words lack semantic duality; there just isn't something else there to name.

If the adverbial theorist concedes the lack of semantic duality in color terms in their ordinary use, how can she explain the nature of the states of affairs that are asserted in (2) and (4) since these are, ostensibly, descriptions of color sensations? Perhaps she will arrive at the conclusion that (2) and (4) are simply false and should be replaced by their true counterparts (2') and (4'). She might also concede that neither (2') nor (4') represent a sensory difference that is introspectively verifiable. Instead she will claim that (2') and (4') are theoretical claims introduced to explain differences in the experiences that we mistakenly describe using (2) and (4). But if the adverbial theory is driven so far from its initial formulations, how are we able to tell what (2') and (4') assert? We have arrived at the point where it is agreed that "bluely" and purplely" do not name anything introspectively detectable, and they do not function semantically in the way that "blue" and "purple" do. So what *do* they designate?

Perhaps they are just dummy terms like variables standing in place of names for the yet to be discovered features that are supposed to explain whatever it is that (2') and (4') are introduced to explain. But what, we may well ask, were they introduced to explain in the first place? Not what (2) and (4) assert because, according to the concessions made by the adverbial theorist, these are false and thus fail to represent anything that needs explaining. So the adverbial theory ends, as far as colors are concerned, as an uninterpreted *explanans* in search of an *explanandum*.

THE METAPHYSICS OF COLOR

In the very first section of *A Treatise of Human Nature*, Hume attempts to establish that "*all our simple ideas in their first appearance are deriv'd from simple impressions...*"[11] Hume quickly recognizes that "there is however one contradictory phenomenon, which may prove, that 'tis not absolutely impossible for ideas to go before their correspondent impressions."[12] This is the famous missing shade of blue which he describes as follows:

> Suppose...a person to have enjoyed his sight for thirty years, and to have become perfectly well acquainted with colours of all kinds, excepting one particular shade of blue, for instance, which it never has been his fortune to meet with. Let all the different shades of that colour, except that single one, be plac'd before him, descending gradually from the deepest to the lightest; 'tis plain, that he will perceive a blank, where that shade is wanting, and will be sensible, that there is a greater distance in that place betwixt the contiguous colours, than in any other. Now I ask, whether 'tis possible for him, from his own imagination, to supply this deficiency and raise up to himself the idea of that particular shade, tho' it had never been conveyed to him by his senses? I believe that there are few but will be of the opinion that he can; and this may serve as a proof, that the simple ideas are not always derived from the correspondent impressions...[13]

On Hume's view, then, not only can one be led to realize that there is a shade of blue that he has never experienced, but he can brought to form a mental image of that very shade. Let us add to Hume's thought experiment the condition that nothing has ever actually exemplified that missing shade; no object ever possessed that shade of blue. Then, the question is: what is the metaphysical status of the missing shade? If we accept the principle that a property exists only if it is exemplified, then we must deny that the missing shade exists.

But should we accept that principle? One argument in its favor is that a necessary metaphysical condition on existence is that something exists only if it enters into the causal order, only if it plays an indispensable role in providing causal explanations of events and states of affairs. Because only exemplified properties play a causal role, only they exist. But why should one want to impose that condition on existence? An argument that might be thought to favor it is suggested by the causal theory of knowledge which says that a necessary condition for something to be knowable to us is that it be capable of entering into a causal relation with our organs of knowledge. Thus anything that lacks causal efficacy can never be known to us and cannot be a candidate for incorporation into our system of existents.

There are, however, well known difficulties with the causal theory of knowledge. We can sometimes have knowledge of the future by inductive inference, and yet these future facts, because they do not yet exist, cannot be causally responsible for our present knowledge of them. We can know truths about numbers, and yet numbers have no causal efficacy. Or consider the case at hand. I can come to know that there is a missing shade of blue and can even form a mental image of it even though that shade by itself is incapable of entering into causal linkages with my sense organs or brain.

Let us suppose that the shades of blue that are observed in Hume's thought experiment are numbered starting with B_1 and that the missing shade occurs between B_{15} and B_{16}. Let us use "B*" as a label for the missing shade. We can formulate the result of Hume's experiment by saying that there is a shade, B*, that comes between B_{15} and B_{16}. But doesn't this formulation, because it is a truth beginning with the quantifier "there is" show that the missing shade exists and that the requirement that only exemplified properties exist is mistaken? Unfortunately, not that much can be squeezed out of the phrase "there is." It is not always used in the existential sense; for instance: "There is a character in *Through the Looking Glass* named Humpty Dumpty" doesn't commit us to the existence of Humpty Dumpty. What is needed is a formulation that starts with "There exists..." We require the existential sense of "There is..."

Perhaps an unexemplified quality such as B* should be considered not as an existent but as a mere possibility.[14] If it should be exemplified, then it is no longer a mere possibility but becomes an existent, something actual. But what does it mean that it itself is a mere possibility? Of course, it is true that it is possible that something exemplifies B*. The table on which I am writing this is white, but it might have been painted with paint of the color B*. All that shows, however, is that that this table has the color B* is a possible state of affairs; there is no law of logic or of nature that prevents B* from being exemplified by the table, that prevents B* from being combined with the table by way of exemplification. But that fact no more requires B* to be a mere possibility than it requires the table to be one. In fact, one would think that if it is possible that certain entities are combined in a certain way, then those entities must be more than mere possibilities. The possibility lies in the combination, not in the items combined.

There is another requirement that is suggested by the causal condition on existence but which leads to a more extensive ontology. It says that we are entitled to accept into our ontology any entity which is indispensable in explaining any fact whose reality we have good reason to believe in. Here explanation is not limited to the causal sort, but includes any sort which we find useful. Thus if we accept that it is a fact that $7+5=12$, and we explain the nature of this fact by claiming that it includes the number 5 as a constituent, then we are thereby committed to the existence of the number 5. Here we explain something not by specifying its causal antecedents—there are none in this example—but by specifying the entities which compose it. Someone who does not want to include the number 5 in his ontology may argue that there is no such fact or that even if there is such a fact, the number 5 is not a constituent of it. No matter how the argument comes out, it is n argument about what is necessary to explain certain facts, given that there are such facts.

It seems that there are certain acts whose explanation makes reference to colors without regard to their being exemplified. Consider (2) and (4) above. That something looks blue to me is one fact; that something else looks purple is another. These facts differ in the thing that appears, but they also differ with respect to the colors that appear. Yet neither implies that the colors are exemplified. So it looks as if we are justified in including colors in our ontology without regard to their exemplification. Of course, if someone can show that the difference between (2) and (4) can be explained in some other way or that there are no such facts whose difference needs to be explained, then our ontology will not include B* for example.

To conclude this somewhat indecisive discussion, what I am inclined to accept is that in visual sensing, one is directly conscious of an array of qualities and relationships. These qualities and relationships are visually presented or given. They are constituted and combined so as to make us believe that they are exemplified as qualities of and relations among physical things. But that they are presented does not entail that they are exemplified. Nevertheless, they are full-fledged members of our ontology. There really is a quality such as B*.

This conclusion can be bolstered by the theoretical advantages that it implies. In the first place, the difference between (2) and (4) can be explained without supposing that there is any semantic duality in the meaning of color terms. The term "blue" means the same whether it is being used to designate a color that is exemplified or one that is merely presented without being exemplified. In the second place, it accounts for their difference without the need to introduce sense data and thus without the attendant difficulties about the nature of mind that sense data carry in their wake.

Some may object that this solution to the problem of visual sensing comes at too great a cost. With respect to colors in particular and visual qualities in general, it commits one to the existence of universals, that is, of a type of abstract object which is capable of being exemplified. And if that is not bad enough, the type of realism about abstract objects to which one is committed is not the modest Aristotelian kind according to which universals exist only when exemplified but the implausible Platonic variety according to which abstract objects form a realm of being that is capable of existing independently of the particulars and individuals which happen to exemplify them. A major objection is that one cannot literally be acquainted with exemplified abstract objects. How can the physical and physiological processes that underlie sense perception bring it about that one can be directly conscious of universals? We understand how it is that we can perceive particulars; perhaps in perceiving particulars we can even perceive qualities that are exemplified. But how in the world can we become acquainted with a quality that nothing possesses or that no particular in the visual field possesses?

These questions are certainly good ones and raise real difficulties for the theory under consideration. However, they derive their force from a certain nominalist prejudice which consists in taking it for granted that particularity and concreteness and individuality are intelligible and need no explanation; the real problem, the nominalist assumes, lies with generality and abstractness, and this is what needs explanation.[15] However, from the realist perspective adopted here, particularity is a greater problem than generality. After all, the entities we are acquainted with are universals—properties, qualities, relations, and so forth. Universals are given, and our consciousness of particulars is mediated by a direct consciousness of universals. Moreover, take any particular and strip it mentally of its properties and relations; there is or seems to be nothing left to account for its particularity. The thing seems to be nothing but the union of the universals which we predicate of it. It seems to me more reasonable to suppose that it is particularity that needs explaining, and that the explanation is going to take the form of an ontology in which abstract objects are indispensable for understanding the nature of particulars.

Russell once remarked that we should not reject a theory of the nature of physical objects just because it strikes us as strange. "The truth about physical objects *must* be strange."[16] Similarly, the truth about perception must be strange. Even for a nominalist it must be strange. If the nominalist accepts that in sense perception certain physical events cause certain sensory events which subsequently lead us to form beliefs and judgments about the world, he is accepting something of which we have no adequate understanding. The basic facts about the interaction of mind and body, facts about sensory consciousness and intentionality, are utterly mysterious; we have no reason to suppose that the truth about these matters, if we should ever come upon it, will comport easily with our everyday understanding of how the world works. Since the causal theory of knowledge is unacceptable, we cannot insist upon a causal condition on the objects of acquaintance. Thus even though it is puzzling to understand how there can be acquaintance with unexemplified qualities, there seems to be no convincing argument that there can be no such acquaintance. And acquaintance of this sort is no more puzzling than the fact that we are able at will to form a mental image of Hume's missing shade of blue.

NOTES

1. John Locke, *An Essay concerning Human Understanding*, Book II, viii, 19.
2. Wilfrid Sellars, *Science, Perception and Reality* (London: Routledge and Kegan Paul, 1963), p. 26.

3. Edmund Husserl, *Ideas Pertaining to a Pure Phenomenology and to a Phenomenological Philosophy*, trans. F. Kersten (The Hague: Martinus Nijhoff Publishers, 1983), p. 91.
4. Wolfgang Kohler, *Gestalt Psychology* (New York: Mentor Books, 1959), chapter 3, especially p. 53.
5. Philippe Brau, Thomas R. Scaiscia, Lynette Linden, and Jerome Y. Lettvin, "The Colors of Things," *Scientific American*, September 1986, p. 84.
6. *Ibid*. p. 87.
7. John Dewey, *The Philosophy of John Dewey*, ed. John J. McDermott (Chicago: University of Chicago Press, 1981), p. 245. For a systematic defense of Dewey's version of naive realism, see his "A Naturalistic Theory of Sense Perception," reprinted in his *Philosophy and Civilization* (New York: Capricorn Books, 1931).
8. *Ibid*., p. 89.
9. *Ibid*.
10. Probably the original presentation of the adverbial theory is contained in C.J. Ducasse, "Moore's Refutation of Idealism," in Paul Arthur Schilpp (ed.), *The Philosophy of G.E. Moore* (La Salle, Illinois: Open Court, 1942).
11. David Hume, *A Treatise of Human Nature*, ed. L.A. Selby-Bigge (Oxford: Clarendon Press, 1985), p. 4.
12. *Ibid*., p. 5.
13. *Ibid*., p. 6.
14. This is the view of Charles Sanders Peirce. "The quality of red...is simply a peculiar positive possibility regardless of anything else." See his *Letter to Lady Welby*, ed. Irwin C. Lieb (New Haven: Whitlock's Inc., 1953), p. 8.
15. Locke, for example, begins his discussion of general terms by laying down the nominalist dictum: "All Things, that exist, [are] Particular." The remainder of the chapter is an attempt to explain linguistic generality without bringing universals into the picture. *An Essay concerning Human Understanding*, III, iii, 1.
16. Bertrand Russell, *The Problems of Philosophy* (New York: Oxford University Press, 1959), p. 38.

CHAPTER 6

COLOR OBJECTIVELY CONSIDERED

PRIMARY AND SECONDARY QUALITIES

In the previous chapter, color was considered in its subjective aspect as an appearance. Now we shall consider color in its objective aspect as a feature apparently possessed by bodies and regions of space. We originally focused upon color because considerations of its status as an appearance suggested interesting differences between visual and other forms of perception. In this chapter we shall discover that reflecting upon color will reveal interesting differences between our common picture of nature and a rival picture that has a better claim to be true.

Philosophers and scientists of the seventeenth century who thought about color and other sensible qualities in the light of the new atomic theory of nature that was beginning to replace the physics of Aristotle had difficulty fitting color into the picture of nature they were then constructing.[1] The entities that the atomic theory postulated in order to explain the observable features and regularities of bodies were understood to be minute atoms or corpuscles that are too small to see with the instruments then available. Each atom was supposed to possess certain intrinsic features such as that it is spatial or extended, that it has a particular shape and size, that it fills space (Locke calls this solidity or impenetrability), and that it is capable of motion and rest. In the terminology that Locke employed, these are the primary qualities of bodies. The other qualities such as color, sound, temperature, odor, and taste are secondary.[2]

There were differences of opinion about which qualities were to be included in each category. For example, gravity did not appear as either a primary or secondary quality on any of Locke's lists, but in his preface to the second edition of Newton's *Principia*, Roger Cotes argued that gravity is a primary quality:

> Since, then, all bodies, whether upon earth or in the heavens, are heavy, so far as we can make any experiments or observations upon them, we

> must certainly allow that gravity is found in all bodies universally. And in like manner as we ought not to suppose that any bodies can be otherwise than extended, movable, or impenetrable, so we ought not to conceive that any bodies can be otherwise than heavy....In short, either gravity must have a place among the primary qualities of bodies, or extension, mobility, and impenetrability must not. And if the nature of things is not rightly explained by the gravity of bodies, it will not be rightly explained by their extension, mobility, and impenetrability.[3]

In this passage, Cotes imposes two conditions on any quality if it is to qualify as primary. First, it must be present in all bodies; second, it must play an indispensable role in explaining "the nature of things." We can see that the list of primary qualities was intended to be complete in the following sense: The explanatory apparatus that consists of the fundamental particles of matter together with their basic features is necessary and sufficient for explaining all physical occurrences and changes.

The apparatus was also used (by Hobbes and Locke, for example) to explain certain mental occurrences, such as the ways in which objects appear to the senses. As Locke says: "it must needs be some exterior cause, and the brisk acting of some Objects without me, whose efficacy I cannot resist, that produces those *Ideas* in my Mind, whether I will or no."[4] That physical changes could produce mental changes and mental changes physical was widely though not universally accepted. Berkeley and Malebranche, for example, thought that direct interaction between mind and body is impossible. However, how matter produces thought was generally believed to be inexplicable by reference to natural forces. As Locke says: "Matter, *incogitative Matter* and Motion, what changes it might produce of Figure and Bulk, *could never produce Thought.*"[5] For Locke, the explanation of the interaction between mind and matter must ultimately refer to the mystery of God's power. Thus there are limits to the applicability of the apparatus of mechanical explanation. Once one brings mind into the picture, different explanatory principles are required.

The debate over whether gravity should be added to Locke's list of primary qualities shows that the very notion of a primary quality—a universal property of matter that is indispensable to the explanatory program of physics—relativizes any given list to the physical theory in place at the time. The correct list of primary qualities can be derived from the correct physical theory. But the list that we have on hand at any period of time is derived from the physical theory believed to be correct at that time.

COLOR AS A SECONDARY QUALITY

According to this mechanical conception of explanation, there is no reason to suppose that any individual atom or corpuscle has a color. It would be superfluous to ascribe color or the other secondary qualities to the individual atoms because color plays no causal role whatever. For example, color would have no influence on the motion that one atom would cause in another by impact. In addition, there is no reason to suppose that the atoms have color in order to explain color appearances. That a tomato looks red, for instance, does not depend upon the colors of the atoms of which the tomato is composed; it does depend upon the effects of the atoms reflected from its surface upon the human eye. Locke thought that the primary qualities of the atoms are sufficient to produce any phenomenal outcome. Therefore, the principle of simplicity in theory construction argued against ascribing colors to the atoms.

To adapt an argument of Locke's,[6] if I should prick my finger with a pin and feel a sharp pain, there is no need to suppose that there is a pain in the pin to explain why my encounter with it caused me pain. The pain is a subjective effect of the pin upon my flesh, not an objective feature of the pin or of any of the atoms that compose it. Apparent color is the same case as pain. That this looks red to me here and now is an effect of its interaction with my visual organs. It is as absurd to ascribe the color I see or am directly conscious of to the object or its atoms as it would be to ascribe pain to the pin or its atoms.

Take two colorless atoms and place them side by side. There is no reason to suppose that the entity which is the sum of both atoms has color if they individually lack it. The explanatory apparatus of atoms and primary qualities has no room for color to arise in this way. Add a third atom and a fourth; the result is the same. The mechanical system of explanation provides no way by which color could suddenly emerge as a property of a group of contiguous atoms if it is not possessed by the individuals of the group. Of course, as the group increases in size, sooner or later it will become visible. But even then there is no need to suppose that the apparent color is a real property of the object; it is a feature that simply appears as a consequence of the effects of reflected light. At no point do we need to suppose that the object really has the color that it looks to have. It may be that apparent color is an emergent quality of the brain-mind system of the perceiver; the introduction of mind brings new principles into play; but nature in itself, independently of the brain-mind system cannot produce apparent color according to Locke's mechanical philosophy.

When I look at the tomato, it looks red, and I acquire the belief that it is red. Is that belief false? That all such beliefs are false, that no belief ascribing a color to an object is true seems incredible and absurd. Call this view *color skepticism*. (To anticipate the outcome of this chapter, this is the view that I will actually defend.) But Locke was not a color skeptic; he was not inclined to adopt a view that is so radically at variance with our common sense, with what everyone believes. The mechanical theory seems to lead to color skepticism, but Locke tried to block this outcome by making a distinction between color as it appears, i.e. the sensation or idea of color, and color as it belongs to objects. That the tomato is red can be interpreted as a true statement provided the tomato has the power to cause a sensation of red in the minds of those who look at it. According to Locke, color objectively considered is not a real quality of bodies as are the primary qualities (it is not, as we would say today, an *occurrent* quality), but a "mere power" to cause certain sensations.

We can formulate Locke's view in the following way. The statement:

(1) The tomato is red.

is true when and only when it is also true that:

(2) The tomato has the power to produce a sensation (or idea) of red in (i.e. to look red to) normal human perceivers under standard conditions of illumination.

What is the relation between (1) and (2)? Locke's view implies that (2) cannot be interpreted as an analysis of the meaning of (1). Although colors are "nothing but powers," nevertheless "they are generally otherwise though of." They "*are looked upon as real Qualities, in the things* thus affecting us."[7] What he means is that we tend to suppose in our every day color judgments that the red that appears and which is in fact an occurrent property of our sensations is also possessed as an occurrent property of the tomato. Our ordinary perceptual judgments make the error of projecting features which exist only as properties of our sensations onto bodies. So when we assert (1), we do not usually mean to imply or assert just (2). We mean to assert that the tomato has a certain occurrent property, not just the dispositional property ascribed in (2). But the assertion we mean to make is mistaken. Only if (1) is interpreted according to (2) does (1) come out true. But (2) fails to yield the intended meaning of (1). The judgment that we intend to make is false, and the one that is true is not the one we intend but rather a substitute for it based upon a certain theory.

This effort on Locke's part to avoid color skepticism does not succeed. Because we project colors onto the world which are not actually there, what we assert in (1) is false. If we interpret our assertions in accordance with (2), what we are then saying is not given by (1) but by:

(3) The tomato is red*.

where "red*" is just an abbreviation of the entire predicate ascribed to the tomato in (2). Thus "red" and "red*" have different meanings and represent different properties on Locke's view. Given what we take colors to be, given our concept or idea of color based upon our experience of colors, red* is not a color at all; it is a power that happens to accompany colors and is founded upon the same primary qualities that cause the occurrence of color sensations. The use of color terms to name secondary qualities, i.e. to name powers or dispositions of bodies, is a philosophical use in which they acquire new meanings and represent a new subject matter. But color skepticism implies that no bodies possess color. To claim that bodies possess color* is not to imply that they possess color. That they possess color* is compatible with color skepticism. Statements about color* are not about color.

THE DISPOSITIONAL THEORY

On Locke's view, (1) and (2) are not semantically equivalent, and that is what drives his position towards color skepticism. But perhaps we should make some effort to avoid his view that our visual experiences and judgments incorporate a projection of color on objects and thus are fundamentally illusory. One way of doing that is just to insist that (2) gives the meaning of (1). As an analysis of (1), (2) tells what colors really are, namely a range of types of dispositions to produce certain sensations. The term "red" in (1) names a disposition of the tomato to appear in certain ways.

However, interpreted in this way, the dispositional theory appears blatantly circular. It is intended to analyse the meaning of "red" as it appears in (1), but the same word reappears in (2). The result is incoherent and uninformative. One way of avoiding circularity would be to adopt a version of the procedure examined in the previous section, in this case by supposing that the occurrence of "red" in (2) is really a different term than its occurrence in (1). To mark the difference replace the "red" in (2) by "red#." Then we replace (2) by:

(3) The tomato has the power to produce a sensation (or idea) of red# in (i.e. to look red# to) normal human observers under standard conditions of illumination.

We require, then, an interpretation of the meaning of "red#" that both avoids the circularity and that shows that its meaning is not the same as that of "red."

The adverbial theory would have been a good candidate for such an interpretation if we had not had good reason to reject it in the previous chapter. In fact the difficulty with the adverbial theory, namely that the "red" in "is red" and "looks red" have the same meaning, that there is no semantic duality as the dispositional theory, taken as a meaning analysis, requires, shows that any interpretation of (3) will fail.

But there is another way of looking at the dispositional theory different both from Locke's and from (3). Consider:

(4) Colors are dispositions of bodies to produce certain visual sensations in humans and other organisms that possess the sense of sight.

There is, on the surface, no circularity here. There is no attempt to provide a meaning analysis of statements ascribing particular colors to bodies. (4) just says what colors are. A critic might suggest that there is an implied circularity contained in the phrase "certain visual sensations." For what are these sensations if not those described by the use of color terms as in "looks red" and "looks green?" I think that this criticism is correct, and the discussion of the previous chapter about the nature of visual sensation confirms that this is so. However, an advocate of the dispositional theory may very well reply that there are features of our visual sensations other than those represented by such phrases as "looks red" that serve to individuate them; perhaps we have no terms in our language for these features just as have no terms to characterize all the phenomenal features of sensations of taste or smell. The advocate may continue by claiming either that phrases such as "looks red" really do not describe our visual sensations at all, or, if they do, there are other individuating features that they do not capture.

Before we pursue the dispositional theory any further, we shall introduce another account of color, the microstate theory.

THE MICROSTATE THEORY

Although most of Locke's statements about secondary qualities characterize them as powers (or dispositions) and not as real qualities as are extension, shape, etc., there is a passage which articulates a different view:

> Thus observing that the bare rubbing of two Bodies violently one upon another, produces heat, and very often fire it self, we have reason to think that what we call Heat and Fire, consists in a violent agitation of the imperceptible minute parts of the burning matter: Observing likewise that the different refractions of pellucid Bodies produce in our Eyes the different appearances of several Colours; and also that the different ranging and laying the superficial parts of several Bodies, as of

> Velvet, watered Silk, *etc.* does the like, we think it probable that the Colour and shining of Bodies, is in them nothing but the different Arrangement and Refraction of their minute and insensible parts.[8]

According to this passage, the secondary qualities are not powers but occurrent features of bodies that produce sensations in the minds of perceivers. These occurrent features are not among immediately observable characteristics of bodies but consist of various relations among their "minute and insensible parts." I shall use the term "microstate" for such characteristics of bodies. In the eighteenth century, Thomas Reid developed this microstate theory in some detail as we saw in our earlier discussion of the perception of heat.[9]

The microstate theory of color can be formulated by:

(5) Colors are those microstates of bodies that are causally responsible for the reflection and emission of waves of light that produce certain visual sensations in humans and other organisms that possess the sense of sight.

Whereas (4) identifies colors with certain powers, (5) identifies them with the occurrent states that underlie and explain these powers. In both cases, the features of bodies that constitute their colors are picked out by reference to their characteristic sensory effects. In both cases, there stands the problem of identifying and individuating the relevant sensations in a non-circular way. Neither theory claims to provide a meaning analysis of color terms; both attempt to tell us what color is rather than what certain words mean.

A reason why (5) has seemed preferable to (4) to many philosophers is that colors are occurrent rather than dispositional features. Our color concepts are no more concepts of dispositions than are our shape concepts. The way colors are presented to us as filling regions of space, covering the surfaces of bodies, and permeating bodies through and through supports allocating them to the category of actual entities rather than mere potentialities. Moreover, color terms are no more overtly dispositional in meaning than are shape terms. Unlike "fragile," "red" is not explicitly a power term. Even though (5) does not pretend to inform us of the meaning of "red," its overtly non-dispositional character means that there is no tension between the meaning of "red" and the nature of red as there is with respect to (4).

There is, however, an epistemological reason for rejecting (5). Color words are terms for observable entities *par excellence*. If anything is observable, colors are. We just *see* what colors objects possess. But the underlying microstates of bodies are theoretical, not observable. How, then, can they be plausibly identified with the most readily visible features of bodies?

Perhaps, however, there is no sharp contrast between theoretical and observable entities. In the very first chapter, we noted that there is a distinction between unqualified and qualified seeing, between seeing something with the naked eyes and seeing something with the use of an instrument. Instruments extend the reach of our senses. An entity postulated by a theory at one time may become observed in the qualified sense if an instrument is developed that is capable of bringing it into view. We also saw then that our eyes themselves should be considered instruments of observation; seeing something with the naked eyes is seeing something by means of an apparatus whose nature and effects themselves need to be investigated. The naive realism of common sense becomes implausible once we look at perception from this perspective. Even unqualified seeing can be interpreted as qualified once we recognize that our eyes are themselves instruments, so although the distinction is embedded in our common sense view, it is not especially fundamental.

Another point deserves mention in this context. In our discussion of the perception of heat, we recognized that we may perceive something whose nature is not manifest via perception alone but requires additional theorizing to produce the proper understanding. Even though I can feel the heat of the stove, observation fails to make the nature of heat comprehensible to me; for that I must turn to thermodynamics. Perhaps these point allow the microstate theory to insist that color is to color perception as heat is to heat perception. We observe it; we see it; but seeing it fails to reveal its true nature; for that we need to turn to color science. We need to distinguish between the manifest and the occult features of perceptible objects. A manifest feature is one that we are directly acquainted with in unqualified seeing. An occult feature is not an object of direct acquaintance even though it may be observable. So the microstate theory says that colors are observable but, like heat, they are occult rather than manifest. The example of heat shows that the very same item is both theoretical and observable; these categories are not contraries at all; color is also, says the microstate theory, both theoretical and observable. So appealing to the perceptibility of color fails to refute the microstate theory.

THE CONCEPT OF COLOR

Each of the two accounts of color that we have been examining claims to reveal the nature of color by telling us what type of entity colors are identical with. That there are entities of these types—dispositions and microstates—is not now in question. What is in question are the identification claims.

If it should turn out that both of these identifications are mistaken, then these accounts are examples of changing the subject. If, for example, colors are not microstates, then discourse about microstates is discourse about a different subject-matter than discourse about colors. However, there has been a certain skepticism of late about whether the notion of changing the subject is sufficiently well defined to be applicable in disputes of this sort. For example, Davidson has argued "that there is no clear line between changing the subject and changing what one say on an old subject."[10] If one takes this skepticism seriously, one may come to believe that there is no objective fact of the matter about what colors really are. Do (4) or (5) tell us what colors really are or do they change the subject? If the case of color falls within the area where there is no clear line, then there is no way of telling which identification is correct. One just say what is useful or convenient to say as the occasion warrants.

A different sort of skepticism about the problem of color takes the line that the issue is a verbal one. What one identifies color with depends upon how one has decided to use color terms. It's up to us what colors are. This perspective is suggested by the following remark of Malebranche's:

> Only since Descartes do we respond to these confused and indeterminate questions, whether fire is hot, grass green, sugar sweet, and so on, by

> distinguishing the equivocation of the sensible terms that express them. If by heat, color, flavor, you mean such and such a movement of insensible parts, then fire is hot, grass green, sugar sweet. But if by heat and the other qualities what I feel near fire, what I see when I see grass, and so forth, then fire is not hot, nor grass green, and so forth, for the heat we feel and the colors we see are only in the soul.[11]

Malebranche asserts that color terms are equivocal; sometimes they denote microstates of bodies, a "movement of insensible parts," and at other times they denote the colors we are directly conscious of in vision which Malebranche thinks reside in the soul. From this point of view, the answer to the question of the nature of colors is that it depends upon which type of entity one chooses to apply color terms to.

We have already seen, however, that color terms in their ordinary use lack the semantic duality that Malebranche's view depends upon. In their ordinary use, color terms appear to represent a definite, identifiable subject matter accessible to the naked eyes and not two or more distinct sorts of subject matter. Of course, a person may decide to use color words to denote dispositions or to denote microstates or denote anything else for that matter. The issue that we are investigating here, however, is not the verbal one of what one is to use color terms for under the condition that there are no prior semantic constraints on their use. Rather, the semantic constraints on their ordinary use point to a definite, visually accessible type of entity that they designate. The issue is to characterize that type of entity and to determine its ontological status.

We are able to specify in a direct way the subject matter our discourse is about because, just as we can point to bodies, we can also point to various of their visible features such as their shapes and colors. Imagine someone saying, while pointing in the direction of the setting sun: "Just look at that color; what a beautiful red." Colors are items of which we are directly conscious; we can see them as well as the objects that exemplify them. When I feel the heat of the stove, what I am directly conscious of are the sensations in my fingers and their discernible features; when I see the color of the sunset, I am directly conscious of it. So the analogy between the perception of heat and of color breaks down. Heat is an occult feature; color is manifest. Whereas the very occultness of heat requires that we call in the help of science to reveal its nature, color is a phenomenal given whose nature is comprehensible by anyone with the sense of sight.

Of course we need the help of science to understand many things about color: its causes, its effects upon the visual system and so forth. But we do not need science to help us determine which items we are studying when we study the colors of things. Because we know directly which items we are investigating in color science, we are in a position to raise questions about *their* causes and *their* effects and *their* ontological status.

Thus the question whether colors, that is, whether these very features of things are identical to dispositions or to microstates or to something else is not the verbal question whether certain words can be used in this way or that. It is a question whether these very features of things are identical with this or with that. There is, then, a fairly clear distinction in the case of color between saying something new about a given subject matter and changing the subject. If, for example, colors, those very things, are indeed the same as the relevant microstates of bodies, then saying so is saying something new about an old subject matter. Of course, the fact that colors are phenomenal and manifest rather than occult is certainly a good reason for rejecting the microstate account. If they are not microstates, then using color terms to denote them would indeed be a case of changing the subject.

THE MEANING OF COLOR TERMS

The first definition of "red" printed in *The Concise Oxford Dictionary* if "Of or approaching the colour seen at least-refracted end of spectrum, of shades varying from crimson to bright brown and orange, esp. those seen in blood, rubies, glowing coals, human lips, and fox's hair." It is perfectly possible that one who knows the English language well-enough to know what "red" means and to be able to use it in a wide variety of situations and to describe a certain range of shades of color knows nothing of the spectrum or of refraction and perhaps has never seen blood or rubies or foxes. It is clear that whatever the definition communicates, it does not specify precisely just what a fluent speaker of English knows just in knowing the meaning of "red." It tries to communicate which color red is by mentioning a variety of items and examples associated with the color in the expectation that the user of the dictionary has had enough experience to figure out the meaning for himself.

The reason why the dictionary approaches the meaning in this indirect fashion is because the quality that "red" represents is what Locke called a simple idea; it is not completely decomposable into component qualities for which we have names. Of course, red is a color; the definition mentions that. It differs from other hues in definite and recognizable ways, but we have no terms in our language to represent these differentia except such descriptions as "the way red differs from green" or "the way blue differs from yellow." Thus what a speaker of English knows when he knows what "red" means is not something that he can perspicaciously and directly communicate in other terms. At best, he needs to use the indirect methods that the dictionary employs.

But then what does he know when he knows the meaning of "red"? In its use as a color word, "red" can perform a variety of functions. For example in "x is red" it is an adjective that functions as a predicate for the purpose of describing something's color. In "x is not red" it is also an adjective used this time to deny a color of something. In "This is a red book" it is an adjective that modifies a noun and tells us the color of the item that the noun designates. In "Red is a color" it is a noun that simply names a particular hue. What all these uses have in common is that "red" stands for a certain hue. So a speaker of English knows which color it stands for in knowing its meaning. That is what knowing its meaning amounts to.

Something else needs to be said to complete the story. Suppose the chair in my study is red. Then the phrase "the color of the chair in my study" when uttered by me stands for the same color as "red." Yet the phrase does not mean the same as "red" even though on occasion it has the same reference. The phrase informs us of the color indirectly; it picks it out by ascribing to it a feature—being exemplified by the chair in my study—that no other color possesses. But it does not tell us which color it is. A person who is ignorant about the chair in my study will still not know what color it has upon hearing the phrase "the color of the chair in my study." Although the phrase stands for the color red when I use it, it fails to express which color it is that it stands for. On the other hand, "red" not only stands for red, it is capable of being used to communicate which color it is that it stands for.

Another way of putting this point is to say that the phrase represents a color via an accidental feature of the color. Since the chair might not have been red, then the color red might not have had the feature of being exemplified by that chair. It is possible that the chair is yellow and that the color of the chair is yellow, but it is not possible that red is yellow. The term "red" designates the color it mean directly without first alluding to any of its accidental features.[12] So one who knows what "red" means knows directly the color represented, a knowledge unmediated by inessential background information. Because red is a simple quality, one comes to know the meaning of "red", one comes to have this direct grasp of the quality meant in virtue of having been acquainted with presentations of red in one's visual experience.

MEANING AND ESSENCE

We already have sufficient reason for rejecting both the dispositional and microstate accounts of color. We are now in a position to provide some additional reasons. We shall focus upon formulations (4) and (5) which are attempts to state the nature or essence of color, what colors are without implying anything regarding the meaning of color terms. This separation of meaning from essence seems plausible for some terms. For example, a speaker of English may very well know the meaning of "water" in the sense of knowing how to use it properly and thus knowing the conditions constraining its proper use without knowing what water is; for that we need to turn to the scientific story to learn that water is a substance composed of H_2O.[13]

Similarly, it might be claimed that one could know the meaning of "red" in the same sense of meaning without knowing the nature of red; for that one needs to turn to the scientific story. However, such a claim is not compatible with the account of meaning given in the previous section. Our everyday pre-scientific knowledge of the meaning of "red" is knowledge of which color "red" stands for and this is a knowledge of red itself unmediated by any accidental or contingent attributions. Thus one who knows what "red" means knows the nature of that color; he knows what color it is; he knows its essence. I do not mean to imply that he can provide an account of its essence in words as one can give an account of the essence of water by saying that it is a substance composed of H_2O. Since it is a simple quality, there is no possibility of a non-trivial verbal characterization. He knows what red is in virtue of having been acquainted with instances of it, of being able to recognize new instances, of being able to distinguish it from other colors, of being able to refer to it and speak about it directly, of being able to imagine instances of it at will, and so forth. He is able to display his knowledge of what it is by means of a variety of intellectual operations directed at the color itself. However, the microstate theory implies that one who knows the meaning of "red" in virtue of knowing English without recourse to the additional characterizations provided by science does not know what red is. According to the account of meaning that I have given, he does know what red is; the scientific characterization provide additional contingent information about red such as that it is caused by certain microstates capable of reflecting light of certain wavelengths and so on.

That this additional information is contingent and not information about the nature of red can be seen by considering this thought experiment: it is logically possible that a change in the human visual system may bring it about that those very microstates and waves of light that now cause a sensation of red cause a sensation of a different color, say a sensation of yellow. Now a sensation of yellow is an appearance of yellow, that is, a presentation of an instance of yellow. In that possible world, that very microstate would, according to the microstate theory, be identical to yellow, not red. So its association with red is accidental or contingent.

Now only can the same microstate underlie different colors in different possible worlds, in the actual world different microstates underlie the same color. We know this from color science; we know, for example, that the same yellow appearance can be produced by various mixtures of light waves. How could the same color be identical with different physical states? That seems to be a logical impossibility. It is much more plausible to suppose that the different physical states are related to the color as causes to an effect; there is no impossibility in different tokens of the same event type having different causes.

How does "red" compare to "water"? Is it the case that we can separate meaning and essence with respect to "water" but not with respect to "red"? Let us imagine that the people living on the shore of a certain lake believe that the liquid that fills the lake is water, their belief being based on the fact that the liquid is perceptually indistinguishable from water on the basis of ordinary unstudied interactions with it. Suppose, however, that a scientific test reveals that it is not composed of H_2O but has an entirely different constitution, say, XYZ.[14] Is it correct to say that this stuff is water, nevertheless? If we say that it is not water simply on the ground that it is not H_2O, that seems to amount to taking being H_2O as essential to being water.

The issue here, it seems to me, turns on the basis of classification that we decide to employ. Let us suppose that we discover that the molecular constitution of various substances is found to correlate with and to explain many fundamental interactions of substances with one another. The molecular constitution is the most important causal fact about substances, so that the theory of molecular constitution becomes one of the fundamental theories for the understanding of physical nature. That would provide a reason for using molecular constitution as the basis for the classification of substances. On these suppositions, which are in fact correct, we could say that the stuff made of XYZ is not really water despite appearances to the contrary. Does that mean that H_2O gives the essential nature of water? That depends upon what you take essence to be. by the real essence of bodies Locke meant the underlying atomic constitution that accounted for the appearances. On his account, then, H_2O would be or be part of the real essence of water. But if by "essence" you mean a property that a substance has essentially independently of any human decision, then, H_2O would not be the essence of water, since the claim that is what water really is founded upon a decision, well motivated no doubt, to employ molecular constitution as the basis of classification.

I do not, however, think that decision plays an analogous role with respect to "red." If we found, for example, that different instances of perceived red were caused or explained by totally distinct types of microstates, we would not think that they were not all reds; we would just say that the same reds can have different causes. The reason is that color is such that what we learn by acquaintance is decisive for determining its nature.

COLOR AND CAUSATION

An argument for the microstate theory can be founded upon the causal theory of perception (CTP), and we shall examine it in this section. The CTP makes the conceptual point that the perceived object necessarily makes a causal contribution to the occurrence of the appearance or sensation which is itself necessary for the perception. It says that it is necessary that only if y appears in some way to x and only if y plays a causal role in the occurrence of the appearance does x perceive y. The CTP must be distinguished from the scientific story which does ascribe a causal role to many of the objects of perception; however, the scientific story is an empirical discovery whereas the CTP claims to be knowable by conceptual analysis.[15] Although they are logically independent of one another, the scientific story can be relied upon to explain the nature of the causal mechanisms whose existence is entailed by the CTP.

The argument goes like this. Consider the red chair in my study; I see both the chair and its color; both the chair and the color appear to me in some way. Since the color appears to me, it must play a role, according to the CTP in the causation of the sensation. But, according to the scientific story, the only factor in the object relevant to the production of the sensation is the microstate that determines which light is reflected and which light is absorbed. There is nothing else for color to be except this reflectance state. So by combining the CTP with the scientific story, we are, so it seems, forced to the conclusion that colors are reflectance states. So the microstate theory is true.

This argument presupposes that the CTP is a correct analysis of the concept of perception. I think that it may be correct in some cases, and not in others. There is no reason at the start to assume that all the perceptual modalities are alike with regard to the causal concept. Take the perception of heat, for example. In order for me to feel the heat of the hot stove by touching it with my finger, it is necessary for me to have a sensation in my finger. If my finger were anaesthetized, then, even if it were in contact with the stove, I would not feel its heat. Not only must the sensation occur when I touch the stove, it must occur as a result of my touching the stove. The heat itself must contribute to the production of the sensation. All this seems intuitively obvious and supports the CTP as applicable to the perception of heat.

But the CTP is less plausible when applied to sound. When I hear the violinist playing, she makes a sound with her violin. The making of a sound is a causal notion, and so the CTP seems correct with respect to the hearing of the source of a sound. But what about the hearing of the sound itself? In order for the CTP to be applicable here, the very sound itself must make a causal contribution to the sensation of sound. But what could that contribution be? The sound itself does not make a sound. In hearing a sound, I apprehend it; I become conscious of it; our concept here is not a concept in which the sound itself does anything or makes any contribution to the hearing of it. Earlier, in chapter four, I argued that the sound itself is internal to the sensation of sound; we discover that by arguments based upon the scientific story; the relation between sound and sensation is not one between cause and effect but one between a constituent and an experience which contains the constituent. I do not doubt that the occurrence of sound sensations has a causal explanation; the point merely is that the sound itself is not one of the causes; it is part of the effect.

A similar account applies to color. According to our concept of seeing, when I see the red color of the chair, it appears to me in some way. I have a certain color sensation, a sensation of red if the perception is color-veridical. To have a sensation of red is just to be conscious of the red color that is presented to me when I observe the chair. There is no implication of a causal transaction between me and the color or between the color and the presentation of the color to me. Our concept of color consciousness is not a concept which includes the idea of the color acting to cause its own appearance. It is not the concept but the scientific story that includes the idea that color experiences have a causal explanation. So one cannot use the CTP to argue in favor of the microstate theory.

There is, however, an argument due to Grice in favor of the CTP as applied to vision.[16] Here is my version of it. It involves the following thought experiment: Suppose someone is able to stimulate my brain directly in order to cause me to have the same experience that I have when I look at the red chair. It is just as if I am seeing the chair and its color even when I am not actually seeing them. Now, suppose I look right at the chair, while my brain is being simultaneously stimulated. I will then have the experience as of seeing a red chair. If the chair is removed, I will continue to have the experience as long as the stimulation is prolonged. Neither the presence nor the absence of the chair makes a difference to the experience I am having; neither the chair nor its color makes a causal contribution to the experience; the stimulation is doing all the work. The argument asserts that in such a case I am not seeing the chair; since the reason I am not seeing it is that it makes no causal contribution to the experience, the conclusion is that its making a causal contribution is conceptually necessary for the seeing of it.

The argument assumes that the key factor that is missing is the chair's role in the production of the experience. However, there is another way of looking at the matter that is, I think, more plausible. It occurred to me while I was thinking about the fact that I occasionally see spots before my eyes due to bits of protein floating about in the fluid behind my eyeball. If I were to draw 1 tiny spot on the wall and look directly at it at an angle in which it is completely covered by one of the spots before my eyes, I would not be able to see it. The spot before my eyes would get in the way and hide it from view. Let us return to the chair. The experience I am having when my brain is stimulated plays the role of the spots before my eyes. The reason that I can't see the chair is that the images produced by the brain stimulation get in the way; they conceal the chair and its color. According to this way of understanding the matter, there is no implication that the missing causal transaction is what prevents my seeing the chair. The crucial factor is that the images blind me to what is before my eyes. For this reason, I do not think that the CTP is applicable to visual perception any more than it is to the perception of sound. I do not think that our pre-scientific concept of seeing implies anything about causation.

However, one may argue that even if the CTP fails, the causal transaction that is at the heart of the scientific story supports the microstate theory. That story tells us that certain reflectance states of bodies cause light to be reflected or emitted; when the light enters our eyes, we are caused to see color. What else could the color be than these reflectance states? There seems to be nothing else in the object for the color to be identified with. If the color were different from the microstate, the scientific story would find no explanatory role for it to play; it would be redundant. Despite the failure of the CTP, it looks as if causal considerations lead us back to the microstate theory.

COLOR SKEPTICISM

This argument for the microstate theory seems quite compelling, but it does make one crucial assumption that can be challenged. It is true that there would be no plausible account of how bodies could exemplify colors if they were not to be identified with microstates. But one cannot thereby conclude that they are identical to microstates unless one assumes that colors are indeed exemplified by bodies. This assumption has seemed so obviously true to most philosophers who have considered the issue that the question that has been most frequently investigated is not: Are colors exemplified? but rather: What exemplifies colors and what are colors to be identified with? I shall call the position that denies this assumption *color skepticism*. It says that nothing has a color, that nothing is colored, that nothing exemplifies any color at all. The color skeptic does not deny that there are sensations of color, that things look to have color. But he points out that the fact that something appears to have a certain property does not entail that it does have that property, so there is no conclusive argument from appearance directly to reality. The term *color realism* is the negation of color skepticism: it says that something is colored.

Color skepticism must be distinguished from a different view that is easily confused with it, namely that there are no colors at all. I shall label this *color nihilism*. If one assumes that colors exist only when they are exemplified, then color nihilism would follow from skepticism. But in chapter five, I challenged that assumption. I there argued for *color Platonism* that says that there are colors and that it is possible that nothing has a color. So color skepticism does not entail nihilism. The view that I think is the most plausible all things considered is a combination of color skepticism and Platonism which says that there are colors and nothing is colored.

I have already said everything I have to say in behalf of Platonism, so the main job in what follows is to defend color skepticism. In the next section I shall sketch the main argument for skepticism. In the next chapter, I will consider a variety of objections to the skeptical position.

THE ARGUMENT FOR COLOR SKEPTICISM SUMMARIZED

One of the main questions of color science is: Why do objects have the colors we see them to have? The structure of the answer has been, since the time of Locke and Newton, that rays of light are reflected and/or emitted from objects, and that the colors we see depend to a great extent upon the particular combination of rays that affect the visual system. Color science attempts to fill in the details of this answer by providing precise characterizations of the physical factors involved including the visual system of the organism. A number of the factors—e.g. light rays, reflectance states, neural processing, etc.—are introduced as theoretical entities justified as the best explanatory hypotheses available at the time.

The crucial fact to note is that colors are not to be found among the factors involved in the explanation of why we see the colors we do. The only place that color terms are actually employed in the explanations is in the descriptions of the sensations caused by the impact of physical energies upon the visual system. But we have seen that this use of color terms is not predicative; to speak of a sensation of red is not to speak of a red sensation. So colored things do not enter the picture at all. But that seems strange for what we began by asking is: Why do objects possess the colors we see them to have? Colors are implicated in the problem to be solved, but once we see the outlines of a solution, we can find no place for color.

Perhaps the difficulty lies not in the solution but in the question. The question presupposes that we see the colors of objects and that objects, therefore, have the colors we see them to have. So let us change the question to: Why do objects look to have the colors they do? Why do we have the color sensations we acquire when we look at objects? The explanations that were given for the initial question apply unchanged to the new formulation. Now colors do not enter the picture at all, either in the explanation or the problem. The scientific story would still hold even if objects never possessed the colors they seem to have.

The color sensations that a given species of animal receives are its subjective reactions to energies impinging upon its nervous system. Different species very likely possess different color sensations, the differences being due to the different ranges of energies their eyes are sensitive to and the different make up of their nervous systems. The explanation of the responses of animals to objects in their environment frequently mentions the color sensations received; that an object of a certain shape looks green to me here and now makes me think that it is a cucumber; since I want a cucumber, I take it. So it is color sensations, not colored objects, that enter into the explanation of animal behavior.

Thus the simplest and most economical accounts of nature and its impact upon mind and action fail to include any ontological commitment to the existence of colored objects. Of course, we all believe in the existence of colored objects; in almost every moment of our waking lives we form beliefs about the color of this and the color of that; these beliefs are involuntary and frequently useful because they track features of objects that may cause us weal or woe. So it is probably impossible for us to become color skeptics in our everyday transactions with objects. However, we are capable of stepping back from our web of belief, of bracketing it, and of asking whether many of the things we are caused to believe to be true really are true all things considered. The considerations just given lead to the conclusion that our color ascriptions are false and our color sensations illusory. Color skepticism is the outcome.

The color realist may reply as follows: "Your argument for color skepticism presupposes first that the explanatory inutility of a type of entity is sufficient to undermine ontological commitment to it, and second that colors cannot be identified with any of the physical factors essentially presupposed in the explanatory scheme of color science. But these presuppositions can be challenged." There is nothing special about the appeal to inutility. Commitments to various types of entities disappear from our web of belief whenever we replace the explanations in which they occur with better ones in which they are absent. "I have no need of that hypothesis," is frequently the best way of dismissing on ontological claim. One who insists upon being a color realist in the face of the argument from inutility is a color fideist as well.

It is true that color realism could be supported by a sound argument that identifies colors with some of the physical factors involved. We have seen that the attempt to categorize colors as dispositions fails because our concept of color is the concept of an actual entity and because dispositional accounts are circular. The microstate identification is more plausible since colors should be entities that bodies possess and bodies do possess the relevant microstates. But the fact that our concept of color is the concept of a directly observable feature of bodies and of space is a strong argument against this approach. Another is that perceived color seems to have properties incompatible with microstates: whereas colors are homogeneous, microstates are not but rather possess a complex internal structure.[17] A third is that different physical states can underlie the same color, so that it is more plausible to suppose that microstates are causes of colors than items that can be identified with colors. A fourth is that the microstate theory, like its dispositional rival, is either explicitly or implicitly circular depending upon the formulation.

I want to mention one last difficulty with the microstate approach based upon an interesting observation of Julian Hochberg's. An instance of yellow may be produced by monochromatic light as in the spectrum, but it may also be produced by mixing together beams of green and red light. In the latter case, the lights do not fuse since the yellow light may be redivided into red and green by passing it through a prism. In general, "lights of different wavelengths can be mixed and separated indefinitely without affecting one another." Hochberg concludes that "when...'red light' and 'green light' add together to form 'yellow,' *the 'yellow' is in us, not in the light, which remains unchanged by the mixing.*"[18] The argument seems to be that since the rays to not fuse and yet we see yellow, not green and red, the yellow we see is not in the light or in the object that reflects light of these wavelengths, but is an effect of the light upon our visual system. We are so made that when we are stimulated by a certain mixture of red and green light, we see yellow. It is not quite right to say that the yellow is in us; what should be said is that we receive a sensation of yellow from the mixture. But once we "subjectivize" certain colors in this way, there is no reason to stop until all colors have been thus "subjectivized." If the yellow from the mixture is just in the sensation because it is an effect of light upon our visual apparatus, monochromatic yellow ought also to be conceived in the same manner.[19]

NOTES

1. See my *Color and Consciousness* (Philadelphia: Temple University Press, 1989), Chapter One for a sketch of the problem.
2. See John Locke, *An Essay concerning Human Understanding*, II, viii for the account of his distinction between primary and secondary qualities.

3. *Sir Isaac Newton's Mathematical principles of Natural Philosophy and His System of the World*, ed. Florian Cajori (Berkeley: University of California Press, 1962), Volume I, p. xxvi.
4. Locke, IV, xi, 5.
5. Locke, IV, x, 10.
6. Locke, II, viii, 16.
7. Locke, II, viii, 24.
8. Locke, IV, xxvi, 12.
9. For Thomas Reid, see his *Philosophical Works* (Edinburgh, 1895), Vol. I, p 313. For a somewhat different presentation of the microstate theory see my *Color and Consciousness*, chapters four and five.
10. Donald Davidson, *Essays on Actions and Events* (Oxford: Clarendon Press, 1980), p. 216.
11. Nicholas Malebranche, *The Search After Truth*, trans. Thomas M. Lennon and Paul J. Olscamp (Columbus, Ohio: Ohio State University Press, 1980), p. 60; quoted in A.D. Smith, "Of Primary and Secondary Qualities," *The Philosophical Review*, April 1990, p. 237.
12. A term that satisfies these conditions is sometimes called a rigid designator.
13. For influential discussions about the relation between meaning and essence see Saul Kripke, *Naming and Necessity* (Cambridge: Harvard University Press, 1980) and Hilary Putnam, "The Meaning of 'Meaning'" in *Mind, Language, and Reality, Philosophical Papers, Volume II* (Cambridge: Cambridge University Press, 1986).
14. This thought experiment has been inspired by Putnam's twin earth example. See "The Meaning of 'Meaning'", p. 223. However, the experiment differs in a crucial way from Putnam's and does not exactly support his conclusion.
15. The classic formulation of the CTP is H. P. Grice, "The Causal Theory of Perception," in *Perceiving, Sensing, and Knowing*, ed. Robert J. Swartz (Berkeley: University of California Press, 1965). There is a certain constraint in Grice's formulation which is relevant here. He says: "The elucidation of the notion of perceiving a material object will include some reference to the role of the material object perceived in the causal ancestry of the perception (or of the sense-impression or sense-datum involved in the perception)." (pp. 438-439) He restricts the applicability of the CTP to the perception of material objects, whereas in our discussion we apply it to certain features of objects such as color and sound as well as to the objects themselves. I see no reason for this restriction since, for example, I sense no difference in the concept of seeing that is exercised in "I see the chair" from the concept that is exercised in "I see the red color of the chair."
16. *Ibid*. pp. 461-462.
17. Wilfrid Sellars, *Science, Perception, and Reality* (London: Routledge and Kegan Paul, 1963), p. 26.
18. Julian E. Hochberg, *Perception* (Englewood Cliffs, New Jersey: Prentice-Hall, Inc., 1964), pp. 20, 22.
19. Additional arguments against physicalistic reductions of color are to be found in Jonathan Westphal, *Colour: Some Philosophical Problems from Wittgenstein* (Oxford: Basil Blackwell, 1987), pp. 67-80. Although physicalistic approaches are often identified with science-based views about the nature of color, this passage by James Clerk Maxwell seems quite compatible with color skepticism: "We are capable of feeling three different color sensations. Light of different kinds excites these sensations in different proportions, and it is by the different

combinations of these three primary sensations that all the varieties of visible color are produced....So far as I know, Thomas Young was the first who, starting from the well-known fact that there are three primary colors, sought for the explanations of this fact, not in the nature of light, but int the constitution of men....Now, if the sensation which we call color has any laws, it must be something in our own nature which determines the form of these laws; and I need not tell you that the only evidence we can obtain respecting ourselves is derived from consciousness. The science of color must therefore be regarded essentially as a mental science." ("On color Vision," in David L. MacAdam (ed.), *Sources of Color Science* (Cambridge: MIT Press, 1970), pp. 75-76.

CHAPTER 7

OBJECTIONS TO COLOR SKEPTICISM

THE PROBLEM OF CONSISTENCY

In this chapter, I will consider a number of fundamental objections to color skepticism.[1] An initial difficulty consists of an apparent inconsistency between the affirmation of color skepticism and the discussion that led up to it. In that discussion, various accounts of what colors are or could plausibly be identified with were reviewed and criticized. In addition, various remarks were made about the nature of color and the meaning of the words we use to talk about colors. It appeared as if that discussion presupposed that there are colored objects, the only question being to understand what that means. It looks, then, as if the assertion of color skepticism undermines the very presupposition of the arguments that were used to justify it.

I do agree that there is an appearance of inconsistency here, but only an appearance. It was much easier to conduct the discussion within the framework of our common sense view of color which, of course, takes color realism for granted. Once, however, color skepticism is introduced and affirmed, the discussion that led up to it needs to be reinterpreted. It should no longer be understood simply as a discussion of what it means for something to be a color and for an object to have a color, but rather as a discussion of our concept of a colored object. We have a concept of color, a concept of a colored object, and common sense accepts that these concepts are non-empty. The argument that leads up to color skepticism can now be interpreted as being about what our concept of color implies about colored objects if there are any. Any statements appearing to presuppose an ontological commitment to colored objects should be reinterpreted so as to cancel any such commitment; they should be interpreted as second order statements about our concepts and beliefs rather than as first order statements seeming to be about colored objects. In this way, the appearance of inconsistency is easily removed.

THE QUESTION OF RELATIVITY

An argument developed by Strawson implies that once we acknowledge a certain relativity in our ascriptions of colors to objects, we will have no reason to be tempted by color skepticism.[2] The argument begins by noting that our ascriptions of properties to objects depend upon our point of view or standard of judgment. For example, from the common sense point of view, the standard we apply is that of "intersubjective agreement," and so we will say that blood is red.[3] From the scientific point of view, the standard we apply comes from physical theory, so we will then be more likely to say that blood is colorless.[4] The affirmation and denial that blood is red can be understood to be consistent "once we recognize the relativity in our conception of the real."[5]

But is blood really red? The only answers available, according to Strawson, are generated by these different standpoints. Can't we ask which standpoint we should occupy to answer the question? But the choice of standpoint is merely a practical issue; there is no fact of the matter to determine that one standpoint is correct and the other incorrect. "We lack reason for saying either that the scientific-objective standpoint or that the human-perceptual-and-moral standpoint gives us the exclusively correct type of conception of the real nature of things. We could have such a reason only if there were a standpoint we could occupy which was superior to either. But there is no such standpoint."[6]

According to the argument, then, the statements:

(1) Blood is red.
(2) Blood is not red.

can be interpreted so as to be consistent with each other. But then how shall we understand them? Perhaps the idea is that they are really shorthand for:

(3) Blood is red from the common sense standpoint.
(4) Blood is not red from the scientific standpoint.

However, it is not at all clear what it means to say that something is (or is not) red from a standpoint. Our concept of color, like our concept of shape, is a concept of a property that objects possess intrinsically; our concept does not suggest that its exemplification is dependent upon or relative to a standpoint.

Strawson identifies a standpoint or point of view with a standard of judgment. So perhaps a better interpretation of (1) and (2) would be provided by:

(5) According to what people agree on using just their eyes, blood is red.

(6) According to what science tells us, blood is not red.

However, this reading fails as an analysis of the meaning of (1) and (2). The standards we happen to use as the basis for ascribing properties to objects seldom or never enter into the meaning of the property words we use. I can assert, for example, that light travels at approximately 186,000 miles per second in a vacuum without having any conception of the method of measurement used in ascertaining the speed of light.

Moreover, although (5) and (6) are consistent with each other, they purchase consistency at the cost of leaving open the very claims that (1) and (2) make. (5) leaves it open whether or not blood is red, but (1) does not. (6) leaves it open that blood is not red, but (2) does not. (5) and (6) allow us to ask which standard we should use to determine the color of blood.

Perhaps the idea is that when (1) and (2) occur in different language games, each may be correct with reference to the rules of the games in which they occur just as "Three strikes, so you're out" and "Two strikes, so you're out" may each be correct in different versions of baseball. In the baseball example, it would be a sheer misunderstanding to ask how many strikes really make an out; so in the color case, it is a misunderstanding to ask what color blood really is. All we have to go on is the language games we play.

However, the various versions of baseball are games in the literal sense, and thus we understand how they can be covered by different rules. But the asserting of (1) and (2) are not literally games or parts of games so it is difficult to understand how they are applications of rules. Of course, one may argue that the meaning of "red" is determined by a semantic rule, but this is, I think, a dubious use of "rule" and a use that fails to clarify how (1) and (2) could be consistent. Suppose I open up a book of color samples and say that for most English speakers, "red" designates the range of colors exemplified on these pages. This claim about the meaning of "red" is factual and empirical and can be supported or refuted by reference to the actual usage of English speakers. One may, perhaps, use this fact to criticize those who use "red" for a different ranges of colors; in that way, the semantic fact about the meaning of "red" becomes the basis for a rule of correct usage. But a rule of correct usage is not itself a semantic fact although it is founded upon one; and it is controversial whether such rules have any binding force at all. And the semantic fact on which it is founded does not provide any comfort to those who claim that (1) and (2) can be rendered consistent.

Strawson's relativity argument is founded upon the premises that different standards that are already in use provide different truth values to the same color ascriptions and that there is no way to determine which standards are correct or which standpoint should be adopted. He thinks that we could evaluate the standpoints themselves only if "there were a standpoint we could occupy which was superior to either." But he doubts that there is a superior standpoint.

The notion of superiority as applied to standpoints is a bit vague. Perhaps all that is meant here is a standpoint from which the other standpoints can be appraised. Now, it is not at all unusual to question and reason about the standards people use in making judgments. There are no 'sacred' standpoints, that is, methods of judgment that are beyond the possibility of criticism. The attempt in philosophy to discover infallible standards of judgment has long ago been abandoned with the failure of Descartes' search for certainty. The absence of a hierarchy of standpoints with an infallible one at the top to be used to appraise all those beneath it does not mean that methods of judgment cannot be evaluated with respect to their reliability, accuracy, and cogency. In such an appraisal, we use other methods of judgment which themselves are subject to possible criticisms. What this means is that there is no infallible termination of the discussion, not that critical discussion is not possible at all. Thus the absence of a superior standpoint in the Cartesian sense does not lead us directly to relativity.

Let me illustrate this in the case of color. Strawson claims that the standard of intersubjective agreement leads us to assert that blood is red. Of course, the notion of intersubjective agreement is a bit vague; it could refer to what many people think, what most people think, what most normal people think, what most people whose faculties are functioning properly think, and so forth. For the sake of the argument, let it refer to what most normal people whose faculties are functioning properly think. And what they think upon looking at samples of blood with their naked eyes is that blood is red.

The first thing to note is that the fact of agreement, even unanimous agreement, does not entail that the belief agreed to is true. There is no inconsistency between "Everyone agrees that P is true" and "P is not true." In the second place, one can rationally reject a proposition that everyone agrees to when their agreement is motivated by factors which are not pertinent to its truth. For example, suppose a group of people plot to murder a certain person and they agree to testify that they saw John Smith commit the crime. A detective as shrewd as Sherlock Holmes would expose their agreement for the sham that it is. They are led to agree by a motive which fails to provide a reason for believing in Smith's guilt. We find agreement persuasive in cases where we think that the circumstances in which the agreement was obtained are indicative of truth. It is the basis of the agreement that is pertinent to the question of truth, not the mere fact of agreement.

We can explain why it is that people agree so frequently in their beliefs about color without bringing color into the picture at all. Their beliefs are grounded on how things appear; the appearances are caused by events that would exist even if nothing were colored. The agreement is driven by the similarities among the sensory effects of objects. So the widespread "intersubjective agreement" is irrelevant to the truth of the propositions agreed to. It would be different if there was reason to believe that the colors that things exemplify actually contribute to the causation of our color sensations; in that case, the sensations would be reliable indicators of color and the beliefs based upon them would have some likelihood of being true. So if color realism was true, we would have some reason to trust our beliefs about color. But the relativity argument was intended to justify a version of color realism by reference to the fact of agreement, whereas the agreement is persuasive of a particular color ascription only under the assumption of realism in general.

Since the argument against color realism in the preceding chapter was based upon the scientific standpoint, Strawson might reply that this case against intersubjective agreement merely begs the question against common sense. Why should we prefer science to common sense when they clash?, he might well ask. The first point to note here is that science and common sense are continuous with one another; they are not totally separate approaches to find out what there is; science is an extension of the more reliable ways of gathering information in ordinary life. Whereas common sense beliefs are based upon casual, sporadic, and unsystematic observations, scientific beliefs are founded upon observations and inferences that are more systematic, careful, precise, and that are better checked and confirmed. Science is epistemically superior to common sense not because it is something totally different but because it is common sense "methodized and corrected."[7] For this reason, philosophical arguments raising doubt about our common sense beliefs that make use of scientific reasonings do not beg the question.

WITTGENSTEIN'S ARGUMENT

In a series of connected passages in his *Remarks on Colour*, Wittgenstein presents a certain account of our color concepts that appear to favor realism. Here they are:

> 96. Because it seems so to me—or to everybody—it does not follow that it *is* so.
>
> Therefore: From the fact that this table seems brown to everyone, it does not follow that it is brown. But just what does it mean to say, "This table isn't really brown after all"?—So *does* it then follow from its appearing brown to us, that it is brown?
>
> 97. Don't we just *call* brown the table which under certain circumstances appears brown to the normal sighted? We could certainly conceive of someone to whom things seemed sometimes this colour and sometimes that, independently of the colour they are.
>
> 98. That it seems so to men is their criterion for its *being* so.

> 99. Being and seeming may, of course, be independent of one another in exceptional cases, but that doesn't make them logically independent: the language game does not reside in the exception.[8]

Wittgenstein accepts that the fact that something looks to be of a certain color and that there is general agreement about how it looks does not entail that it is of that color. He also accepts that the fact that it looks to be of a certain color is a reason for thinking it is of that color. How it looks, however, is not just our evidence for its color; the apparent color is the *criterion* for the real color. In other words, the fact that, for example, something's looking brown is a reason for thinking that it is brown is not founded just on a contingent correlation between looking and being brown; the connection is conceptual or logical or grammatical, even though it is not one of entailment. No appeal to scientific or other facts could show that its looking brown is not a reason for thinking it is brown. Thus our color concepts provide a reason for rejecting color skepticism because, as long as things appear to have colors, we always have a reason for thinking that they are colored.

On the basis of various hints in Wittgenstein's writings, we can construct a powerful argument in favor of his criterial view of color concepts. It goes like this. We have a linguistic practice or language game of calling something brown when it looks brown. There are exceptional cases in which something looks brown but isn't or is brown but doesn't look it. However, our color concepts are constituted for the normal case; the exceptional cases are just that: exceptional. That there are exceptions prevents the connection of seeming with being from being one of entailment. But the very idea of the normal case is itself embedded in our concepts, and this prevents the connection from being merely contingent and factual. There are certain contingent facts which give point to our linguistic practice with color terms, namely that people generally agree on the colors things look to have and on the colors they do have. These facts make it possible to play the game with color concepts; if people did not agree, we would not have the conception of color that we possess. The contingency of these facts, however, is compatible with the conceptual connection between seeming and being.

Moreover, our primary access to the colors of objects is via their appearance. It isn't as if we know, on the one hand, about the colors things look to have, and then, quite independently, discover what colors they do have, and note a correlation between them. If the appearances did not constitute criteria for the reality, we would have no access to the reality at all.

I think that one can accept Wittgenstein's criterial view and still be a color skeptic. Even if looking brown is a criterion for being brown, in any particular case it is a reason which can be defeated by considerations that have greater weight. For example, though something looks brown to all of us in this room, we are all being deliberately exposed to an optical illusion in which things that are red are made to look brown. The fact that a linguistic practice is so constituted that certain concepts are in their very nature reasons in favor of certain judgments does not require that any of those judgments be true.

Color skepticism does not just raise doubts about this, that, or the other color ascription; it raises doubts about all of them simultaneously. Thus it seems to reject the very idea of the normal case embedded in our language game in which seeming and being coincide. Every case becomes exceptional, and that seems incompatible with the concepts we have. Although we can defeat individual color ascriptions for particular reasons, we cannot, the color realist may argue, defeat all of them by a wholesale reason which turns the normal case into the exceptional.

I think that the color skeptic has a perfectly satisfactory reply. The first point to note is that our color concepts do not of themselves specify the factors which explain the exceptional cases. Why seeming fails to coincide with being in this case must be determined by the circumstances and cannot be extracted from the concept. For example, what makes all the red objects in this room look brown to this group of people cannot be specified ahead of time or deduced from the concept of color. Therefore, it is logically possible that in every case there are particular circumstances which defeat the inference form seeming to being. Moreover, we can adopt a perspective from which wholesale failures of the inference seem quite likely. What I have in mind here is bringing other species of animals into consideration whose different visual apparatus makes it quite likely that their color perceptions are significantly different from those of humans. From a biological and evolutionary perspective, color sensations are species specific responses to impinging energies that occur because of their utility with respect to the survival and well-being of the animal. That one such species has developed language games that are based upon the illusion of color realism does not make color realism andy the less of an illusion. Suppose all species that possess the sense of sight developed language games making use of color concepts. While there might be a great deal of intra-species agreement, there would be little inter-species agreement. Which species is right about the colors things really have? This question seems quite senseless; we can avoid species chauvinism by adopting color skepticism and supposing that color perceptions are useful illusions. The conceptual connections embedded in our language game our perfectly compatible with color skepticism provided we see this particular game as a useful device whose utility does not depend upon its mirroring reality. This particular game happens to be infected with our biologically determined projections. Once we understand that, we will realize that in order to obtain a conception of the way the world is, we must learn to discount the peculiarities of human and of animal experience; the psychic additions projected onto the world by our nervous systems must not be confused with the properties that objects really have. Color skepticism is a way of making this point.

EMERGENCE

A color realist may adopt the view—call it *emergent color realism*—that colors are emergent properties of bodies. He can respond to the color skeptic as follows: "Even if you are correct in thinking that colors cannot plausibly be identified with microstates or light waves or dispositions or other candidates drawn from physical theory, that is no bar to there being colored objects. If none of these identifications is plausible, color can still be something in its own right. It can be an emergent property. By an emergent property I mean this: Suppose you have an object composed of parts which have various properties and relations to one another. These properties and relations are features of the parts, not of the object of which they are parts. For example, take a rock whose parts are molecules with various properties and relations specified in physics and chemistry. An emergent property of an object is, first of all, a property of the object rather than a feature of the parts. The rock's gray color is an example. Another requirement for emergence is that the property is not conceptually or logically reducible to the features of the parts. Thus the shape of the rock may not be emergent because if we know all the spatial relations among its constituent molecules, we would then know how they are arranged, and we would thereby be able to figure out its shape. A third requirement is that the object's having an emergent property is to be explained by reference to the structure of its parts. The rock has this color because it has this molecular structure. Thus an emergent property is one that is supervenient on the structure and features of the parts in the sense that things that differ with respect to the property will also differ with respect to its structure and/or features of its parts."

The emergent realist continues: "I agree with your account of the concept of color, and hence I too reject the various identifications that you have criticized. But I would defend the common sense of the matter by claiming that things do have color over and above their physical characteristics. The idea that color is an emergent property is just a technical formulation of what we all believe. Emergent realism is more plausible than color skepticism because it is consistent with the evidence of the senses: we *see* the colors of objects; that there are colored objects is a rock bottom fact whose denial is just unbelievable."

I shall take up the argument from the evidence of the senses in the following section and will confine my remarks here to the topic of emergence. To make it easier to think about the issue, let us consider it in the light of the seventeenth century compuscularian hypothesis on the basis of which Locke made his distinction between primary and secondary qualities. On this view, if you remember, perceptible bodies consist of clumps of atoms each of whose properties are amongst the primary qualities and each of which has spatial, temporal and causal relations to others. Let us imagine someone whose job it is to create a rock by bringing together the atoms with the appropriate primary qualities one at a time. We can understand why the rock comes to have the shape and size and weight it has by reference to the individual atoms, their features, and spatial arrangement. These features are not emergent but are conceptually implied by the features and arrangement of the parts.

When the 'rock-creator' begins his task by bringing together just a small number of atoms, the rock does not yet have its gray color. But when the clump of atoms has reached a certain size and complexity of structure, as soon as the next atom is added, it becomes colored. That it acquires just this color at this time cannot be predicted on the basis of our knowledge of the primary qualities and structure of the parts. That's why color is emergent; it is something completely new that has sprung up when the underlying object is of an appropriate level of complexity.

There are three major difficulties with this notion of color emergence. First, according to the picture of emergence just given, the rock did not have any color when it has only *m* atoms, but it acquired a color upon the addition of the *n*th atom. But that seems unintelligible. How could one or a few more atoms make such a difference? What is there about there being *n* atoms which allows for emergence whereas *m* atoms were insufficient? There doesn't seem any theoretical foundation either in the corpuscularian hypothesis or modern atomic theory for the emergence of colors. Of course, the addition of new atoms does sooner or later make a difference; as the clump reaches a certain size it becomes visible and it seems to us to be gray. This we can explain: its increase in size allows it to reflect enough light to cause our visual system to produce visual sensations. But this story does not require nor does it imply colors as emergent qualities.

Second, emergent colors are both theoretically and practically useless. We can account for all color phenomena such as the appearances of colors, our beliefs about color, the causes of the appearances and beliefs, and so forth, without bringing emergent colors into the explanatory apparatus. They are, at best, epiphenomena, bereft of any causal or explanatory function. They are postulated merely to satisfy a prejudice; that the prejudice is well-entrenched and ineliminatable does not make it any the less a prejudice.

Third, because they are bereft of a causal role, if there were emergent colors we would have no way of knowing it. Since our color sensations are not dependent upon their presence, the sensations would not function as indicators of them. Because they have no explanatory role, we could not infer their reality via an inference to the best explanation. Of course, one may claim that our knowledge of them is grounded upon our seeing them. We shall consider this argument in the next section.

The emergent realist does have an interesting response available to the first difficulty that emergence is unintelligible in the case of color. Consider the sequence of events that begins with my turning the ignition key in my car and ends with its engine starting. One may intelligibly ask how it comes about that my turning the key happens to have this result. The answer is given by providing an account of the intervening events. The turning of the key leads to event *a*, and *a* causes *b*, *b* causes *c*, *c* causes *d*, and so on until we arrive at an event that directly and immediately causes the engine to start. We render a causal sequence intelligible in this way by filling in the gaps. Intelligibility is a product of a certain sort of narrative. The question: "How does it happen that this leads to that?" is in place when we are ignorant of some of the events between this and that.

Now consider two events, *e* and *f*, that are contiguous so that there are no gaps between them to fill. For example, let *e* be a moving billiard ball coming into contact with a second ball; let *f* be the initial motion of the second. Hume pointed out that without reliance upon our past experience of the interaction of objects like billiard balls, we would have no reason to suppose that *e* would cause *f* rather than anything else. *A priori*, anything can cause anything. Because there are no intervening events, we cannot explain why *e* caused *f* by filling in the gaps. To the question "How does *e* cause *f*?" we should answer: "It just does; that's the way the world works." That a pair of contiguous events causally interact is a brute fact susceptible of no further explanation. Explanations come to an end somewhere; that they come to an end in the case of contiguous events is founded upon the fact that there is nothing more to say. When you have contiguous events, it is a mistake to demand an explanation. The only rational response to brute facts is to accept them.

The color realist is in a position to respond as follows: "The reason that the emergence of colors in objects that possess a certain degree of complexity in their underlying structure seems unintelligible is that the emergence is a brute fact. Causal relations can be made intelligible if you have gaps to fill in. But ultimately we come to events that are contiguous, and here it is not possible to render the connection intelligible. The emergence of color is an event of this sort. So the lack of intelligibility is not an objection to color emergence."

"In addition," continues the realist, "I know that you are sympathetic to a certain solution to the mind-body problem which can be called *emergent materialism* according to which some mental events can be identified with brain events that have emergent properties that are constitutive of their mentality. So you are as committed to brute-fact emergence as I am. There is a similarity between the problem of color on the one hand and the mind-body problem on the other. In both cases, various forms of reductionism have failed. Just as it is implausible to suppose that colors are reducible to physical microstates, so it is implausible to suppose that mental properties are reducible to purely physical properties. You are being inconsistent because you countenance emergence in the mind-body case but not in the case of color."

This is a good reply, but it is not sufficient to save color realism. What the reply shows is that the argument from unintelligibility is far from conclusive. But there is an important difference between the color problem and the mind-body problem. Consider the case of pain. When I have a toothache, I am directly conscious of it; I feel it; I am aware of it. The explanation of how I come to believe that I have a toothache makes reference to the fact that I feel it. Thus mental events play in indispensable role in explaining our beliefs about them. That is one reason why eliminativism is implausible in the mind-body case. So we might be willing to accept mental properties as emergent properties both because we cannot eliminate them, and because emergence is the least bad of the available alternatives. But eliminativism is plausible with respect to color just because exemplified color has no explanatory function. Whatever function it seems to perform can be assumed by the physical microstates or light waves or color sensations, etc. So the argument from unintelligibility against color emergence gains strength when it is conjoined with the fact of color's explanatory uselessness.

THE EVIDENCE OF THE SENSES

In the course of defending color skepticism before various audiences, I have found that the most common reaction has been one of sheer incredulity and instantaneous rejection. To the extent that this reaction can be put in the form of argument, it goes like this: "How can you possibly deny that objects have color? We see their colors; nothing is easier to see; nothing is better supported by our sense experience. What better evidence can you have about anything than the evidence of the senses? We have the best possible reason for thinking that the colors we see are really there. Even though your arguments for color skepticism are plausible and convincing, they are not strong enough to outweigh the evidence of the senses. Such evidence is rock bottom. Even if we are unable to reply to your arguments or to diagnose their fallacies, we are assured that they are indeed fallacious and that you are trying to make the worse argument appear the better. In addition, you agree with everyone else that material objects have size and shape; you are not a size skeptic or a shape skeptic. You too rely upon the evidence of the senses. But your use of this evidence is unjustifiably selective. If you judge that the tomato is round on the basis of what you see, you ought also to affirm that it is red on the basis of what you see. As a matter of fact, because you have the best possible reason for thinking that it is red, you *know* that it is red. Thus in affirming color skepticism, you are contradicting things that you know to be true. You are defending a position that is indefensible, and we are rightly convinced, even before you begin your defense, that color skepticism is a lost cause."

In order to assess the cogency of this objection, let us reflect upon the following example. There are people who see spots before their eyes because certain impurities in the fluid behind their eyeballs casts a shadow. Imagine a group of such individuals gathered together in the office of an ophthalmologist waiting to be examined. In speaking to one another, they discover that they agree that the world is spotty. Not one of them disagrees; they see the spots, and they think that they have the best possible reason for believing that the world is spotty.

We know that they are mistaken; the world is not spotty. So they do not have the best possible reason for thinking that it is. Thus the evidence of the senses, even if supported by the agreement of others, is not, *ipso facto*, the best possible reason for believing anything. It is *a* reason, no doubt. It is reason that can be strengthened to some extent by intersubjective agreement. And if Wittgenstein is correct, that it is a reason is not just a contingent matter of fact, but is a 'grammatical' fact embedded in our perceptual concepts. But no amount of intersubjective agreement ever makes it the best possible reason because one cannot exclude *a priori* the possibility of there being evidence that, in any particular case, outweighs evidence provided by the senses.

A reason that we have for thinking that the people who believe that the world is spotty are mistaken is that the world does not appear spotty to us. But why is our agreement to be trusted and their's not? Perhaps the fact that they agree on the evidence of their senses is just as good a reason for them as our agreement is for us. Thus, as we saw earlier, we must go beyond the mere fact of agreement to bring in additional factors.

The relevant factor in this case is that there is something wrong with their eyes. That's why their agreement is not convincing. The world appears spotty to them not because it is spotty but because of the shadows cast by the impurities in the fluid behind their eyeballs. To us, the world appears free of spots because it is free of spots; there is nothing the matter with our eyes that would make actual spots invisible to us. However, their agreement is not based upon sensory appearances whose occurrence is dependent upon the facts that appear; there are no such facts; their experiences are not under the control of a spotty world; that is why they are not veridical. In general, when our experience is veridical and the world appears as it really is, then our experience is under the control of or is dependent upon the facts that appear. In certain cases, we are in a position to establish or to explain failures of veridicality by identifying the causes of the experiences and finding out that these causes have nothing to do with the states of affairs that are thought to appear. Thus, the ophthalmologist is in a position to explain to his patients why their agreement counts for naught as evidence about the way the world is.

We are now in a position to understand why the argument against color skepticism based upon the evidence of the senses fails. We have no reason to suppose on the basis of the scientific story about perception that our color sensations are under the control of or are dependent upon colored objects. Given the makeup of our visual apparatus, we would have just the color sensations we do caused in the way they are usually caused even if there were no colored objects. If we follow out the chain of causation, we do not come upon colored objects. In that respect, we have no more reason for supposing that the appearances of color to us are any more likely to be veridical than are the appearances of the spots to the patients. But this way of looking at the matter also shows why the arguments for color skepticism fail to lead to shape skepticism. Normally the shapes objects actually have play a role in the causation of the shapes they appear to have. If we follow the chain of causation, we come upon shaped objects.

We have an inborn tendency to trust the evidence of the senses. If we were to try to justify this trust, we would discover that it depends upon a presumption that our experiences are mostly veridical. Through experiencing failures of veridicality, we modify the tendency somewhat so that we learn to trust our senses more in some circumstances than in others. Our inborn trust is shaped and modified and qualified by the experience of error and the failures of our expectations and intentions when errors occur. We also acquire the ability to explain the sources of error, and in many such cases, the explanation reaches beyond the resources of common sense and falls within the purview of science. Color skepticism is a result of this process of applying our understanding of the nature of perception to the assessment of the degree to which our experiences are veridical and of the reliability of the evidence of the senses. Thus, we have the ability to use our senses in combination with our rational faculties to develop theories which can then be applied to determine with greater exactness the actual informational content of our sense experience. Our experiences are our reactions to impinging energies, and there is no alternative but to call upon scientific theory to assess what they are capable of telling us about the world that causes them.

NOTES

1. I considered several basic objections to color skepticism in chapter eight of *Color and Consciousness, An Essay in Metaphysics* (Philadelphia: Temple University Press, 1989). The material that follows in this chapter supplements and amplifies those arguments.
2. See P. F. Strawson, "Perception and its Objects," in Jonathan Dancy (ed.), *Perceptual Knowledge* (New York: Oxford University Press, 1988) and *Scepticism and Naturalism: Some Varieties* (New York: Columbia University Press, 1985).
3. Strawson, "Perception and its Objects," p. 112.
4. *Ibid.*, p. 110.
5. *Ibid.*, p. 111.
6. Strawson, *Scepticism and Naturalism*, p. 53.

7. These are Hume's words which he used to describe philosophy. However, in Hume's time, philosophy included what we call science. See his *An Enquiry concerning Human Understanding* (Indianapolis: Hackett Publishing Co., 1983), p. 112.
8. Ludwig Wittgenstein, *Remarks on Colour* (Berkeley: University of California Press), p. 29e.

CHAPTER 8

KNOWLEDGE AND PERCEPTION

COLOR SKEPTICISM AND THE PROBLEM OF KNOWLEDGE

In this final chapter, I shall consider color skepticism to be an established view and shall proceed to discuss some of the epistemological questions it raises. Ancient and modern skeptics have frequently pointed out that our senses are deceptive; failures of veridicality occur that lead us to adopt beliefs that are false. Their arguments are occasionally based on pointing out certain examples of deception such as the straight stick that looks bent in water or the round plate that looks elliptical, and so forth. Texts on the psychology of perception are filled with examples of illusions and hallucinations of one kind or another. But such examples fail to support the case that our senses are radically deceptive.

In the first of his *Meditations*, Descartes began by alluding to examples of this sort, but then developed his dream argument to support the view that our senses are capable of being radically deceptive and thus should not be trusted until considerations are advanced showing that this capacity is not, in fact, realized. What color skepticism shows is that our senses are systematically deceptive in certain respects: none of our visual experiences are veridical with respect to color, and all of the beliefs we have which ascribe a color to an object are false. However, color skepticism does not go as far as Descartes' radical skepticism; his dream argument is intended to show that our perceptual experiences are capable of failing to be veridical in all respects: nothing is as it seems.

The argument for color skepticism is incompatible with radical skepticism. It is an argument that is based upon scientific realism that says that there is an external world with a certain character that affects our senses in various ways and that certain aspects of our visual sensations fail to match or correspond to anything in that external world. The radical skepticism of the dream argument, if it could be established, would undermine the basic principles underlying color skepticism.

Later, I shall return to this topic and consider Descartes' challenge to our pretensions to possess knowledge of the external world. There is, however, a related challenge that lies implicit in the discussion that led up to color skepticism. Earlier I argued against naive realism in favor of a representative theory of perception; a stage of that argument consisted in taking the subjective turn according to which perception is to be understood as an achievement of sorts mediated by inner sense experience. Our perceptual beliefs are based upon this inner experience and are reliable to the extent that it is veridical. But if experience constitutes our only direct access to the external world, and if there is no way of comparing our experiences to the world to determine their degree of reliability, we can, it seems, reasonably raise the question whether our senses are to be trusted at all. The scientific realism that underlies our discussion leads us to the subjective turn that itself raises doubts about the realism. Thus the argument of the preceding chapters is threatened with a fundamental incoherence.

Therefore, it is appropriate at this point to turn to the question whether perception can constitute a foundation of our knowledge of the world. It would seem that perception cannot constitute a foundation because we must appeal to theory to determine the extent of its veridicality; such an appeal leads to color skepticism which refutes the presumption of general veridicality. But, it appears, the very theory that is employed to appraise the pretensions of perception is itself based upon perception. How can the very theory that limits the pretensions of perception be founded upon the very grounds that it criticizes?

In order to achieve a perspective on these issues, some remarks are necessary about the nature of knowledge and about the implications of our conception of knowledge with respect to the question whether we possess perceptual knowledge.

KNOWLEDGE AND BELIEF

Our interest here is in determining whether the beliefs we form based upon sensory information can constitute knowledge. We are thus concerned with the kind of knowledge Ryle called *knowing that* or propositional knowledge in contrast to *knowing how* and other conditions that we use the verb "know" to characterise.[1] Sentences that express *knowing that* assertions are typically of the form:

(1) X knows that P.

where "X" is a variable whose substituends are names or descriptions of particular knowers and "P" is one whose substituends are sentences expressive of propositions. A proposition is whatever it is that can be said to be known in the *knowing that* sense. Whatever it is, it is something capable of being either true or false.

The first issue to be discussed is the question of the necessary and sufficient conditions of (1). We are not interested in constructing a definition for the verb "know" for that has a variety of usages, and probably any definition would just consist of a list of them; in fact, that is what the definitions that actually occur in dictionaries consist of. What we are after is this: consider a situation in which a person makes a claim of the form (1); suppose others are interested in the truth of his claim, take it seriously, and undertake to investigate it carefully. Situations of this sort are typically manifested in scientific inquiry. What general conditions are required for (1) to be true, where the level of generality is so understood as to be independent of the content of any particular substituend for "P"? It is, of course, possible that even the serious and careful uses of (1) that I have in mind are so vague as not to be governed by necessary and sufficient conditions. In that case, what would be wanted is a set of characteristic circumstances which justify the use of (1).

One must be careful, however, in the way we understand the notion of *use* here. One of the uses of (1) is in situations in which the speaker intends to provide assurances to others of the truth of a substituend of "P." The notion of *use* involved here consists of the communicative intention of speakers. However, since people who possess knowledge do not always communicate it and since the notion of *knowing that* does not logically involve communication, reference to the typical communicative intentions governing the use of (1) are irrelevant to the question we are investigating. This point can be marked by saying that what we are after is the semantic, not the pragmatic, conditions for the use of (1).

There is one popular account of the semantic conditions of (1) that I shall label *the standard account*. It says that *knowing that* consists of true justified belief. More formally, it claims that the following three conditions are individually necessary and jointly sufficient for the truth of any case of (1):

(a) P.
(b) X believes that P.
(c) X is justified in believing that P.

There are various versions of the standard account in which different terms are used, but I shall take this version as the basis for discussion.

(a) is the least controversial of these conditions. It is widely accepted that "X knows that P, and P is false" is inconsistent so that (1) entails that P is true. *Knowing that* is like an achievement; when we know a proposition to be true, we have captured a truth. In this way, knowledge is distinguished from belief because you can believe something that is false as well as true.

An apparent difficulty with (b) is that sometimes, so it is said, we use "believe" as a verb of contrast to "know" as in "I believe it even though I do not know it." However, this claim could be appropriate even if "believe" and "know" do not exclude one another; all that is required is that "I believe it" makes a weaker claim than "I know it." Moreover there is no absurdity in asking: "Which of all the things that I believe do I really know?" This suggests that something that I believe could also be something that I know as well.

Another difficulty is based on the fact that the concept of belief is one of a group of concepts—being of the opinion that, thinking that, being sure that, accepting that, agreeing that are some others members of the group—that have similar import. So it seems arbitrary to select belief as the one constitutive of knowledge. What the members of the group have in common is that they represent the acceptance of the truth of a proposition to some degree or other. So we could just as well replace (b) with:

(b*) X accepts that P.

with the understanding that "accepts" represents the various members of the 'acceptance group,' any one of which can enter into particular instances of (1) depending upon the nuance appropriate to the circumstances.

There is an objection that (b*) as well as (b) are too weak on the grounds that one knows that P only when one is sure of it. Thus A. J. Ayer writes: "One is not reasonably said to know a fact unless one is completely sure of it...To say of oneself that one knew that such and such a statement was true but that one was not altogether sure of it would be self-contradictory."[2] According to Ayer, being sure does not consist of a particular mental episode: "It does not seem to consist in any special mental occurrence. It is rather a matter of accepting the fact in question and of not being at all disposed to doubt it than of contemplating it with a conscious feeling of conviction."[3] Ayer would have us replace (b*) with "X is completely sure that P."

For Ayer and other philosophers, *knowing that* requires certainty as a condition. But a distinction here is necessary because two different sorts of certainty are pertinent to the issue. There is the certainty that pertains to me when I say "I am certain" and the certainty that pertains to the proposition when I say "It is certain." I may be certain even when it is not certain, and in that case I have made the error that consists of the strength of my conviction outrunning the strength of the evidence. Let me call the first sort of certainty *subjective* and the second sort *objective certainty*. Ayer's claim is that *knowing that* entails subjective certainty. It entails that the proposition accepted should be accepted with a great degree of conviction.

I think, however, that Ayer's suggestion confuses knowing with knowing that one knows. Suppose that I once learned from a very reliable source that the population of Alabama was over 3,000,000. Although I have forgotten where I learned it, the fact remained at the back of my mind so that I actually still think that Alabama's population is over 3,000,000. However, if I am asked whether I know it, I may feel quite uncertain, and reply that I do not know it but only think so. However, although I lack subjective certainty, my belief has objective certainty since I acquired it from an unimpeachable source that in fact was right. *It* is certain even though I am not certain. Thus I do not know that I know it; in fact, I think that I do not know it. But since even sincere claims about what one knows are not infallible, it is possible that I know it nevertheless. In fact, since it is certain as well as true and accepted by me, our concept of knowledge allows me to say that I really do know it. A person may be confused and unsure about what he actually knows. To deny that means that one is committed to the view that one knows only if one knows that one knows. But that claim leads to an unending regress and hence is absurd.

There is the further difficulty with (b) (that I mentioned in chapter two) that being in a particular mental state, call it belief, opinion, or what you will is not at all necessary for knowledge. In Popper's terms, we are capable of having objective knowledge.[4] Suppose that I have been engaged in research on the demography of Alabama and have recorded the information I discovered in a notebook. If I am asked whether I know Alabama's population, I could very well respond: "I sure do; I have it right here in my notebook." There are various places in which a person can store his knowledge of facts and information. One place is his brain or mind; other places are his notebook, his computer disk, his filing cabinet, his index cards, and so forth. An advantage in storing it in one's brain is that one has access to it no matter where one is; disadvantages are that the space for storage is limited and one does not want to clutter it with unimportant details nor take the time to memorize it. While one knows the things that one remembers, one does not always remember what one knows.[5] Traditional discussions of knowledge have overemphasized the min/brain as a place of storage, and thus have tended to use mentalist terminology to formulate the second condition. To avoid this error, we should interpret (b*) so that acceptance does not entail mental storage. That is another reason for preferring (b*) to (b). In what follows, my use of the notion of belief as a condition of knowledge should be understood in the light of these qualifications.

KNOWLEDGE AND JUSTIFICATION

The main argument for condition (c) in the standard account of knowledge is that one can have true belief or true acceptance without knowledge. One can believe what is true for the wrong reasons. The reasons can be false as when one thinks that a man called Eliot wrote "The Wasteland" on the grounds that it was written by George Eliot.[6] Or the reasons may be true but irrelevant or non-evidential as when one comes to believe that one will certainly pass the examination on the grounds that one dreamed that one will pass it. So it looks as if one knows that P only when the reasons for accepting P are both true and relevant. When one has such reasons, then one is justified or warranted in accepting P. That is how justification comes into the picture. Something more is needed for *knowing that* than just true belief; the term "justification" stands for a family of terms any one of which can be used to stand for this third condition. This term has a wide variety of uses, most of which are irrelevant to the question of knowledge: one can be justified not only in believing certain propositions but in performing certain actions or understanding certain projects or feeling certain emotions, and so forth. Moreover, not every case in which "justified" is applied to beliefs is pertinent. For example, a person may argue that he is justified in believing P on the grounds that he ought to be allowed to believe it without legal penalty; he is here making a political claim that is not relevant to the question whether he in fact knows P. The relevant use of "justification" is epistemic in which that which does the justifying point in the direction of the truth of what is believed.

In an influential paper, Edmund Gettier has argued that even with the addition of (c), the standard account fails to provide a sufficient condition for knowledge.[7] He offers the following as a counter-example to the standard account. Suppose that Smith and Jones have applied for a certain job and, on the basis of strong evidence Smith comes to believe that:

(i) Jones will get the job, and Jones has ten coins in his pocket.

Now, (i) entails:

(ii) The person who will get the job has ten coins in his pocket.

Smith accepts (ii) on the grounds that he deduced it from (i) for which he has strong evidence. Suppose that (ii) is true not because (i) is true and (i) entails (ii), but because, as it turns out, it is Smith, not Jones who will get the job, and Smith by chance has ten coins in his pocket. Not only does Smith believe what is true, but, so it appears, he is justified in his belief because he accepts it on the basis of a proposition which entails it and for which he has strong evidence.

Despite the fact that the three conditions for knowledge on the standard account are apparently satisfied, Gettier claims that Smith does not know that (ii) is true. The reason is that (ii) "is true in virtue of the number of coins in Smith's pocket while Smith does not know how many coins are in Smith's pocket, and bases his belief...on a count of the coins in Jones' pocket, whom he falsely believes to be the man who will get the job."[8]

Gettier bases his argument against the standard account on the assumption that "for any proposition P, if S is justified in believing P, and P entails Q, and S deduces Q from P and accepts Q as a result of this deduction, then S is justified in believing Q."[9] This assumption allows that one is justified in believing Q even if P is false and is a wrong reason provided one has strong evidence for it. In the example, not only is (i) false but it is actually irrelevant to the truth of (ii) despite the fact that it entails it. It was just an accident that Smith arrived at the truth by accepting (ii) on the basis of (i).

I think, however, that Gettier's example is not a genuine counter-example to the standard account. For if the premises on the basis of which one comes to accept a proposition are false or irrelevant, then, even if one is justified by evidence in accepting the premises, one is not justified in accepting the conclusion. What the example actually shows is that Gettier's assumption is mistaken. It fails to provide a sufficient condition for justification; in fact, the very reason Gettier gives for thinking that Smith does not have knowledge is also a reason for thinking that Smith lacks justification. For a necessary condition for justification based upon reasoning from premises is that one not base one's belief upon wrong or irrelevant reasons. The fact that the reasons entail the belief is not of itself very important because for any conclusion, there are an infinity of propositions that entail it.

There is, however, a genuine difficulty with the standard conception. Suppose that I know that the contents of a certain bag consist of 60 red and 40 green marbles. I am told to draw one marble from the bag, but before doing so I am asked to predict the color of the one I draw. If I get it right I will be given a certain amount of money, and I lose nothing if I get it wrong. I predict a red marble, and then draw a red marble. My prediction is true. I am also justified in predicting red over green because there is a much greater chance of a red one being drawn. So it looks as if, assuming that predicting can be equated with accepting, all the conditions for knowledge are satisfied according to the standard account. My prediction is true, and I am justified in it because the evidence that red will turn up is stronger than the evidence that green will turn up. But, obviously, I do not *know* that the marble I will draw will be red.

The problem illustrated by this example is that one can be justified in accepting a proposition that, on the evidence, is very uncertain, the uncertainty preventing one from possessing knowledge. The evidence is too inconclusive for knowledge; although it makes the prediction more likely than not, it does not endow it with sufficient likelihood for it to be a case of knowledge as distinct from true justified acceptance. What is missing is objective certainty. The prediction is not certain because the evidence does not insure or guarantee its truth. If I knew ahead of time that all the marbles in the bag are red, then my prediction would have been a case of knowledge.

We need, then, to modify the standard account in order to avoid such counter-examples. It would be wrong, I think, to require that in the justification, the evidence statement must entail the conclusion or be conclusive in some other way. For that would be to assume that in all cases of *knowing that*, the justification always consists in deriving propositions from other propositions. That assumption would lead immediately to difficulties concerning perceptual beliefs for these seem to be derived not solely from other propositions but from something non-propositional, namely sense-experience. The notion of justification we need should cover cases of both propositional and non-propositional derivation.

The solution that I suggest is simple and modest; in order to have knowledge, not only must the proposition I accept be true, but I must be *fully* justified[10] in accepting it. The term "fully" is intended to exclude those partial justifications as in the marble example that fall short of the certainty required for knowledge.

One might object to the suggestion by saying that the notion of being fully justified is really so vague as to be useless. What makes a justification a full one? The modified standard account says nothing about this. I agree that the modification I have suggested is vague and not very informative, but I think that this is an advantage rather than a disadvantage. The conditions we are after in formulating an account of *knowing that* must be so general as to be independent of the specific content of the proposition said to be known. Since propositions of quite different content will be justified in different ways and will have different conditions of objective certainty, we cannot build these details into the general conditions of knowledge. The basis for my knowledge of mathematical propositions will not be the same as my basis for perceptual or inductive beliefs. Thus the bases for knowledge and justification for particular classes of propositions cannot and should not be built into the general account of knowledge. They belong, rather, to the theories that explain how each of these classes is justified.

So the account of knowledge that will enter into the following considerations is that a person knows that P if and only if P is true, she accepts that P is true, and she is fully justified in accepting that P is true.

JUSTIFIED ACCEPTANCE

Although I shall use the term "justified" and occasionally the term "warranted" for that property of the propositions that one accepts that are necessary for *knowing that*, it must be understood that there are a variety of other terms that play a similar role and that may be more appropriate in certain contexts. It should be understood that a proposition can be justified although false. Of course, if one knows it, then it must be true, but truth and justification are logically independent conditions. I shall use the term "acceptor" for the person or other agent who accepts the proposition whose justification is in question.

It is now necessary to introduce two qualifications into the account of knowledge of the last section. First, justification is relative to an acceptor. To say that a belief is justified is incomplete; one must say to whom it is justified. The evidence available to me may be such as to justify P but the evidence available to you may justify the negation of P. There is no contradiction in saying that P is justified to X at time T and P is not justified to Y at time T. A proposition that is justified to certain acceptors at one time may fail to be justified to anyone at a later time. The available evidence changes, and this requires us to reassess our beliefs. Science is an institution which deliberately creates ways and means for evidence to be made public. Evidence that has entered the public domain may be said to be available to all members of the community of inquirers, or at least to all of those who have access to the relevant documents. When a theory is supported over its rivals by the evidence that has entered the scientific domain, then we can speak simply of its having scientific justification, although this is short for its being justified to the members of the scientific community having access to this domain at the time in question.

Second, we must distinguish *justification to* from *justification for*. For every justified belief or proposition, there is always an acceptor *to whom* it is justified as we have seen. But *justification for* may be absent. In order for a proposition to be justified for an acceptor, not only must it be justified to her, but, in addition, she must also know what it is that is doing the justification. There are cases as I shall soon argue in which a person is justified in accepting P but has no idea what the justification consists in. Ignorance of what justifies is sometimes consistent with being in possession of a justification.

What it is that justifies a belief to someone I shall call its *epistemic basis* or just *basis* for short. Suppose the basis that justifies P to X is B. For example, B might consist of certain true propositions that entail P. In this case, in order for X to be justified, it is not enough that B be thought of or entertained by X. Even if B entails P, X might not have put two and two together; X might have accepted P for some other reason or for no reason. In order for B to justify X in accepting P, it is necessary that P be accepted *in virtue of* its basis B. The phrase "in virtue of" stands for whatever the connection is between the acceptor and basis which is necessary for the basis to succeed in justifying the belief to the acceptor. This connection might differ for different types of bases. From now on, in speaking of the basis of a proposition for an acceptor, I shall assume that the relevant connection holds. I shall use the term "basis relation" for this connection.

Even though truth and justification are logically independent, they are internally related one to another. When B justifies P to X, the relevant epistemic notion of justification is the one that justifies X in thinking that P is *true*. Justification is something that in its own nature points to the truth. It may fail to guarantee the truth because P may be false or because B may be weak and inconclusive. But B must have some property in virtue of which P is more likely to be true than not. How else could X be warranted in accepting P *as true*? I shall call such a property *a truth selector* and shall say that any basis that exemplifies a truth selector *tends toward the truth*.

To illustrate some of these points, let us consider the case of our memory of the occurrence of particular events we have experienced. Suppose X met Y on a certain day and later remembers having met Y on that day. Memory beliefs are peculiar in that they arise in our consciousness in a certain way, we are able to classify them as memories, and yet, unless we are neuro-scientists, we have no idea of the nature of the underlying mechanism that causes them to persist and become conscious. Let us suppose the mechanism consists roughly of this: X's experience of meeting Y left a trace R in his brain. In certain circumstances, this trace is activated and causes him to think that he met Y. The basis of X's memory belief is R; R exemplifies a truth selector, namely the property of being caused by the very event that makes the belief true. X is justified in his belief that he met Y. That belief is justified *to* X; but it is not justified *for* X, because he has no understanding or knowledge of its basis. Since the basis R guarantees the truth of the belief, X is fully justified in believing that he met Y, and therefore, he knows that he met Y.

Instead of introducing the concept of a truth selector as I have done, some philosophers prefer to speak of a reliable process. X is justified in his memory belief because it is based upon a reliable process, one that produces truth more often than not. Remembering is a reliable process because the traces that underlie it are more often than not caused by the events said to be remembered. However, I prefer the truth selector approach, because it is logically possible that there are particular cases that embody truth selectors which justify even though these cases cannot be generalized to a repeatable process. Perhaps the truth selector is exemplified only once. However, when the truth selector is a property that is repeatable, then the truth selector approach approximates the reliable process approach.

JUSTIFICATION AND FAITH

I mentioned earlier that the concept of justification has a variety of uses, most of which are not pertinent to the condition of knowledge we are after. In order to enlarge upon this these, I shall here consider a possible objection to this account of epistemic justification that is based upon the point of view expressed in William James' essay, "The Will to Believe."[11] James is concerned to argue against the view that it is wrong to believe or to accept a doctrine on insufficient evidence. He was concerned to legitimize religious belief even in those cases where the evidence was not sufficient to support it. He thought that in certain circumstances, "our passional nature" can legitimately determine our beliefs instead of evidence.[12] In general, these circumstances occur when the belief is such that its truth or falsehood cannot be decided by reference to evidence and when believing it makes an important difference to our lives. He thought that a person might very well be justified in believing in God, for example, even though he could not support his belief by argument or by reasoning. Using my own terminology here, we can put the point by saying that according to James, a person can be justified in believing P even when there is no basis for his belief.

Because of the various uses of "justified," there need not be any inconsistency between James' view of religious belief and the view of justification I have argued for. Under the topic of faith, philosophers and theologians have attempted to formulate general conditions under which people are permitted to believe some things, obligated to believe others, and forbidden to believe still others. Here is an insightful passage from Locke that bears upon this issue:

> There is no Body in the Commonwealth of Learning, who does not profess himself a lover of Truth: and there is not a rational Creature that would not take it amiss to be thought otherwise of. And yet for all this one may truly say, there are very few lovers of Truth for Truth's sake, even amongst those, who perswade themselves that they are so. How a Man may know whether he be so in earnest is worth enquiry: And I think there is this one unerring mark of it, *viz.* The not entertaining any Proposition with greater assurance than the Proofs it is built upon will warrant. Whoever goes beyond this measure of Assent, 'tis plain

> receives not Truth in the Love of it; loves not Truth for Truths sake, but for some other end. For the evidence that any Proposition is true (except such as are self-evident) lying only in the Proofs a man has of it, whatsoever degrees of Assent he affords it beyond the degrees of that Evidence, 'tis plain all that surplusage of assurance is owing to some other Affection, and not to the Love of Truth....Whatsoever Credit or Authority we give to any Proposition more than it receives from the Principles and Proofs it supports itself upon, is owning to our Inclinations that way, and is so far a Derogation from the Love of Truth as such: which as it can receive no Evidence from our Passions or Interests, so it should receive no Tincture from them.[13]

Locke is here arguing that a person who loves truth for its own sake and has no other purpose in mind in his inquiries should believe only on the evidence (putting aside self-evident propositions) and should adjust the strength of his belief to the strength of the evidence. Locke's rule is that belief should be proportioned to and controlled by the likelihood of its being true. To the extent that it is measured by any other standard, the acceptor has some other motive than the love of truth for its own sake.

In the chapter on enthusiasm from which this passage is drawn, it becomes clear that Locke is not just expressing his own preference for the love of truth for its own sake but thinks that it would be wrong, perhaps morally wrong, to engage in inquiry for any other purpose. "*Reason*" he says "must be our last Judge and Guide in every Thing." Otherwise "every Conceit that thoroughly warms our Fancies must past for Inspiration, if there be nothing but the strength of our Perswasions, whereby to judge of our Perswasions; If *Reason* must not examine their Truth by something extrinsical to the Perswasions themselves; Inspirations and Delusions, truth and Falsehood will have the same Measure, and will not be possible to be distinguished."[14] And even more strongly, if our beliefs are not controlled by reason, that is, by the evidence, we place our selves "in the power of the Prince of Darkness."[15] It becomes clear from the tone and content of this chapter that for Locke it is not optional that reason control our inquiries; it is a moral imperative.

The issue between Locke and James is ultimately ethical. Is a person morally permitted to determine his beliefs (to the extent to which it is in his power to do so) by considerations that do not aim at truth? On Locke's view, one is morally justified in believing only those propositions that are also epistemically justified and only to the degree to which they are epistemically justified. For James, occasionally, one is morally justified in beliefs that fail in epistemic justification or that outrun their epistemic justification. This is not an issue that it would be appropriate to pursue here. I wish only to make the point that we need to distinguish the question of epistemic justification from ethical and other value considerations about what is permitted, obligatory, and forbidden. To point out, for example, that a person's belief outruns the evidence on which it is based or is not based on any evidence at all is not to say that she has made a mistake or done anything wrong. It is just to say that the belief fails to be epistemically justified. To claim with Locke that epistemic considerations alone should control the existence and strength of belief is to make an ethical rather than an epistemological evaluation. The latter is concerned solely with the appraisal of the relation between the grounds of acceptance and the likelihood of truth.

KNOWLEDGE AND CERTAINTY

Not all warranted beliefs count as knowledge because some of them are false. But not all those that are true are cases of knowledge either. My expectation that the next marble I draw will be red, though correct (here I am ignoring color skepticism and speaking with common sense in order to preserve the example), is not knowledge because its basis is not strong enough; a probability of 60% does not provide the degree of certainty required for knowledge.

What degree of certainty is required? There is some agreement that 70% is not enough, nor is 80% or 90%. What about 99%? If I know that 99 marbles are red, do I know that the next one will be red? Here people tend to disagree; some feel intuitively that the probability is sufficient for knowledge, others that only 100% will do, and still others feel that the whole issue may now be a verbal one to be settled by stipulation.

I am among those who think that only 100% will do. Suppose that the bag held 100,000 marbles 99% of which are red. That means that 1000 marbles are green. If there were one million marbles, 10,000 would be green. That's a lot of green marbles. There is nothing here that guarantees the truth of my prediction. It is only when 100% are red that it becomes certain that the next one will be red. The truth selector must be one that guarantees truth in order for knowledge to be possible.

A skeptic might argue that even in the 100% case I do not have knowledge. Suppose that I know that every marble in the bag is red but perhaps the one that I pull out turns green as it comes into view. Isn't that possible? If so, it isn't certain that the next one will be red. However, the skeptic's point is mistaken. Suppose she is correct that it is logically possible that the marble will turn green. But that is irrelevant. Though possible, it won't happen. In fact, the red one I select will continue to be red. That's how things work in our world. The basis does not have to guarantee truth in all possible worlds, just in this one, the actual world.

Perhaps the skeptic intended to refer not to logical possibility but epistemic possibility. Perhaps she means that for all I know, the marble will turn green. Is that right? Don't I know that a change in a material object's spatial position is not of itself sufficient to modify its color? Don't I know that no red to green color changing events are present to turn the emerging red marble green? But let us put all this aside and give the skeptic the benefit of the doubt. (Of course, skeptics seldom give anyone else the benefit of the doubt.) Let us suppose that for me it is epistemically possible that the next marble will not be red. Suppose I say: "It is possible, for all know, that the next marble will not be red as it comes into view even though I know that all the marbles in the bag are red."

Even so, it seems to me that I do know that it will be red. After all, the basis guarantees that it will be red, whether I know it or not. Perhaps I do not realize that it is certain that it will be red because I am ignorant of certain facts about the world. Perhaps I will even say that I do not know that it will be red. I may accept that it will be red; I may even accept that my belief is warranted, and yet, convinced by the skeptic's appeal to epistemic possibility, deny that it is certain that it will be red. But it is certain whether I realize it or not. I know that it will be red even though I do not know that I know it. In order for me to know that I know it, I must know that all the conditions for my possessing knowledge are satisfied. But the requirement for full justification, for certainty, for a guarantee may indeed be satisfied without my realizing it. I may think that my justification is weaker than it is. We are not infallible in our assessments of the strength of the grounds of our acceptances, and thus we are not infallible in our classifications of our cognitive achievements.

UNDERSTANDING AND INSIGHT

Suppose a perfectly reliable mathematician point to a proof written in a language that I do not understand and says that it proves the truth of the proposition expressed by the last line of the proof. Let "S" stand for the sentence that constitutes the last line. What I know as a result of the guarantee I have received is that there is some true proposition expressed by "S." Do I know the truth of the proposition expressed by "S"? How can I? I do not even know which proposition it is.

Let "T" stand for the translation of "S" into English. I neither understand the meaning of "S" nor do I know its English translation. So it cannot be true that I know that T. Now someone may argue against this as follows: You do know the truth of the proposition expressed by "S." You have a guarantee of its truth from a perfectly reliable mathematician. That proposition is the very one that is expressed by "T." Of course, you do not know that it is expressed by "T," and therefore you are not in a position to acknowledge the truth of "I know that T." But whether you acknowledge it or not, it is true nevertheless. There is a description "the proposition expressed by 'S,'" and you know that the proposition that satisfies that description is true. There is another description of the same proposition, "the proposition expressed by 'T'" which you are unfamiliar with. But one does not need to know every description of a proposition in order to possess knowledge of it; one is enough.

This objection is mistaken because it assumes that all descriptions are equal as far as knowledge is concerned. For me to know that there is some true proposition that satisfies a certain description is not sufficient for me to know that that very proposition is true unless the description is one that tells me which proposition it is. It must be a description by means of which I am enabled to *understand* the proposition. Understanding is another necessary condition for knowledge. Understanding is necessary for my belief or acceptance to latch on to the right propositional content.

Understanding is frequently a matter of degree. The schoolboy who has memorized a geometrical theorem which he has written down in his notebook at his teacher's dictation has less of an understanding than he later will when he can prove it on his own and less again than he will when he sees it as a part of a wider mathematical system with its relations of implication to other propositions within the system. Let me use the term *insight* to represent what the schoolboy gradually acquires as he comes to see the theorem in its wider logical and geometrical context. The schoolboy at first had knowledge without insight; when he is able to prove it on his own, he has acquired partial insight which becomes fuller as he acquires greater mastery of the system as a whole. A minimal understanding is necessary for knowledge, but one can possess knowledge without having much insight. The possession of knowledge can be a rather superficial affair, and it frequently is.

Knowledge is not necessary for insight. Given the conception of knowledge for which I have argued, one that involves certainty and a guarantee of truth, it is doubtful that most of our currently accepted scientific theories count as knowledge. Even if we are justified in accepting them, our evidence is seldom strong enough to guarantee their truth. Nevertheless, people are capable of grasping these theories with different degrees of insight. The process of education is in part one of increasing the student's insight into and mastery over various subject matters.

Bases of justification vary in the degree of insight they provide. Consider again the example of the schoolboy who has memorized the theorem dictated to him by his teacher. Let us assume that the teacher is perfectly reliable and has never assured anyone of the truth of a theorem that wasn't true; let us also assume that his reliability is not accidental but is based upon his own mastery of the subject he teaches. The schoolboy thus has a guarantee of the truth of the theorem, and he can be said to know it. His basis is the teacher's word which exemplifies a perfectly reliable truth selector. However, this way of acquiring knowledge conveys almost no insight. While the teacher's word is a basis that fully justifies acceptance, it fails to convey any understanding of why the theorem is true. It is a reason for believing but not a reason for the belief. I can have a reason for thinking *that* something is true that utterly fails to provide any insight into *why* it is true. Even if education must begin by employing such superficial though reliable bases as the teacher's word, it must move on by teaching bases that provide insight and thus mastery over subject matter.

NON-PROPOSITIONAL JUSTIFICATION

Suppose X met Y some time ago and now remembers it and knows that he met him because of his memory. In order for this memory to emerge into his consciousness, certain physiological and psychological conditions must be satisfied; for example, there very likely has to be a brain trace, and certain events have to occur to activate it. In addition. X must possess those conceptual abilities that are necessary for to him to be able to articulate the judgment that formulates the content of his memory. But if we try to identify the basis for the judgment, it is very likely that we will not come upon anything propositional. The trace is activated, certain brain events ensue, and X judges that he met Y. There is no inference here of the judgment from other judgments. We have here a wholly non-propositional basis and wholly non-propositional justification. In contrast, if X is convinced of the truth of a theorem T solely as a result of his deducing it from the axiom set A all of whose members are self-evident for him, then we here have a wholly propositional basis and wholly propositional justification.

Some bases are mixed. For example, suppose that X met Y sometime ago; at that time Y was already an old man and was suffering from a number of serious diseases. Now X concludes that Y is dead. His conclusion is based on his recollection of the meeting and of the age and condition of Y, but it is also based on a premise that someone that old and that ill has not very long to live. So the non-propositional memory basis combines with certain background beliefs to produce this result. The background beliefs are essential to justify the conclusion.

A *basic belief* is one that has a wholly non-propositional basis. A belief that has a wholly propositional basis or a mixed basis is *derived*. Some of our beliefs may have no bases at all and fail to be justified; these are our *prejudices*. People usually think that their prejudices are justified and are frequently willing to cite evidence for them. But since what they cite as evidence fails to justify, it does not count as a basis. I shall call the *grounds* of a belief whatever it is that is a person's reasons for accepting it. Some grounds are bases but, when the belief is a prejudice, its grounds do not constitute a basis. A prejudice that has no grounds is a basic prejudice; if it has grounds it is derived.

FOUNDATIONS

Are there any basic beliefs? Until the development of coherence theories of truth and knowledge in the Hegelian tradition, most philosophers thought that there must be. Consider as an example Hume's view. There are two kinds of objects of human knowledge, relations of ideas and matters of fact. Mathematical knowledge consists of relations of ideas, and every such proposition known to be true is either self-evident or deduced from self-evident propositions. According to Hume, "propositions of this kind are discoverable by the mere operation of thought, without dependence on what is any where existent in the universe."[16]

Those that are known by deduction are, in our terminology, derived and have a wholly propositional basis. Those that are self-evident or "intuitively...certain"[17] are basic beliefs; our knowledge of them is not based upon deriving them from other propositions. They have a basis that they exemplify which, for lack of a better phrase, I will call *direct certainty*. Hume took it for granted that direct certainty is a perfectly reliable truth selector, one that provides a guarantee and that can serve as a basis for knowledge. Your may recall that Descartes in the third *Meditation*, was troubled by direct certainty or by what he called clear and distinct perceptions; he wanted to know how we can be sure that ideas that are clear and distinct are indeed true. To dispel any residual doubts he undertook to prove that there a God who is not a deceiver. Whatever one thinks of his argument, his great achievement here was in raising the question and showing the difficulty of answering the skeptic who wonders whether some alleged truth selector is really truth tending. The problem of legitimizing appeals to direct certainty was of less significance to Hume because he thought that knowledge of the relations of ideas does not provide any insight into anything that exists. He put more effort into analyzing our knowledge of matters of fact or "real existence" and argued as follows that such knowledge is founded upon basic beliefs which are representations of sense perception and memory:

> If we proceed not upon some fact, present to the memory or senses, our reasonings would be merely hypothetical; and however the particular

> links might be connected with each other, the whole chain of inferences would have nothing to support it, nor could we ever, by its means, arrive at the knowledge of any real existence. If I ask, why you believe any particular matter of fact, which you relate, you must tell me some reason; and this reason will be some other fact, connected with it. But as you cannot proceed after this manner, *in infinitum*, you must at last terminate in some fact, which is present to your memory or senses; or must allow that your belief is entirely without foundation.[18]

The process of giving reasons cannot continue indefinitely; sooner or later it will terminate, if it leads to knowledge, in some state of affairs that is given; if the state of affairs is past, it is given to memory, if present, to the senses. Hume showed great insight in placing memory on a par with the senses. After all, any fact that is given via sensation quickly becomes past and remains accessible only through some trace that it leaves such as a memory trace.

Implicit in this passage is the standard argument against a pure coherence theory of knowledge, namely that unless our reasonings possess some link to the world via perception and memory, our beliefs about matters of fact could never constitute knowledge or even be justified; they would be purely hypothetical. There are many possible internally consistent sets of beliefs; these beliefs purport to refer to matters of fact independent of our belief systems. A belief about a matter of fact is true only if the matter of fact which it represents exists, so justification must somewhere involve a linkage to the world. In creatures such as us the basic linkage consists of sense experiences and their traces left in memory. Moreover, it is implied by Hume's argument that the ultimate foundation of our knowledge of matters of fact must be wholly non-propositional. For suppose it is mixed; then its basis consists of some proposition together with some sensation and/or memory. But then what is the basis of that proposition? Sooner or later we must arrive at a sensation or memory if it is to be justified. Thus propositions formulating our sense-perceptions and memories are the basic beliefs which, for Hume, constitute the sole foundation of human factual knowledge.

Before considering certain arguments against Hume's view of the foundations of knowledge, some distinctions are in order.

PERCEPTUAL JUDGMENTS

A *perceptual judgment* is a report one makes to oneself or others of what one takes oneself to have seen or heard or felt or otherwise perceived through the senses. A *sensory judgment* is a report of one's sensations, of how things appear. There are mixed judgments which mention both what is perceived and how it appears, as in "The banana looks green."

Perceptual judgments when properly grounded upon sensations are capable in principle of counting as knowledge. They are grounded upon sensations either directly or indirectly. Indirectly when they are conclusions derived from sensory judgments as would have occurred if Macbeth had inferred from the judgment that it seems to him as if he were seeing a bloody dagger to the conclusion that there really is a bloody dagger that he is seeing. Directly when they are grounded upon sensations without the intervention of a sensory judgment.

There is an argument that says that perceptual judgments can never be justified by reference to sensations or sensory judgments alone but always require in addition the use of background knowledge or information. How can one be justified in concluding that something is green on the basis of its looking green unless one makes use of the additional premise that things of this sort that look green usually are green? According to this argument, the pattern of justification of a perceptual judgment requires there to be a sensation with or without a sensory judgment together with a background belief that provides a reason for thinking that the sensation is veridical. Without such a reason, it is claimed, the sensation may constitute a ground of the judgment but never a basis for it. The conclusion is that the position that Hume argues for must be wrong; whatever the role of sensation is in the justification of perceptual belief and judgment, it cannot provide the sole epistemic basis as Hume implied. Background information is always indispensable to pass from sensation to the external world.

The error in this argument is the claim that the background belief is indispensable as far as justification is concerned in the passage from sensation to judgment. Suppose I have a sensation which is such that it seems to me as if I were seeing something yellow. Suppose it also true that more than half of the time when a person has a sensation of this sort, there really is something yellow that is being seen. Then the sensation exemplifies a truth selector, and since the sensation triggers the judgment that there really is something yellow that I am seeing, it serves as a basis that really justifies the judgment. It is not required as far as justification is concerned that the proposition (H) that more than half of the time when a person has this sensation, there really is something yellow there plays a role in the triggering of the judgment; all that is required for me to be justified is that H be true, because its truth is what endows the sensation with a truth tending truth selector. It is not necessary for H to be a part of my background beliefs at all.

The defender of the argument may reply that without the presence of H in my background. I would have no reason to make the perceptual judgment that I do; I would never have arrived at the judgment. What reason could I have for thinking that this sensation indicates the presence of a yellow object unless I believed H? The sensation itself won't trigger the judgment without H being engaged in the process.

Now this last point may very well be true, but it does not serve to support the original argument. It is necessary to distinguish between what is necessary for the justification of a judgment and what is necessary for its formation. Even if the presence of H in the background is necessary for the latter, it does not follow that it is required for the former. Many conditions of a physiological and psychological sort may be necessary for the formation of a judgment; these are *motivating conditions*. But not every motivating condition plays a role in the basis.

In addition, it is not obvious that the presence of H in the background is even necessary as a motivating condition. When I come to think that I am seeing something yellow on the basis of having a sensation of yellow, I am not sure that H is part of my background. Perhaps my brain is programmed to generate the judgment automatically given the sensation. After all, our perceptual judgments are for the most part involuntary and out of our control; there is seldom any conscious and deliberate consideration of premises in the process generating thought from sensation. That H is an indispensable motivating factor is a psychological claim whose truth or falsehood does not affect the epistemological claim that the sensation serves as a basis whether H is present in the background or not.

PERCEPTUAL KNOWLEDGE

Under what conditions does a perceptual belief or judgment count as knowledge? When the sensation that triggers it exemplifies a truth selector that guarantees its truth, that makes it objectively certain. Here are two examples of such truth selectors. The first is when the particular sensation is perfectly reliable, when it is a sensation of a type all of whose instances are caused by the state of affairs represented in the judgment. For example, if I believe that this is round because it looks round, and if every case of something's looking round is caused in the right way by something's being round, then the truth of the belief is certain and I thereby not only believe it but also know it.

A second is when the occurrence of the sensation is not accidental, when it looks round because it really is round, when its looking round depends on its being round, when it would not have looked round were it not for the fact that it is round. The first type of truth selector—perfect reliability—is also an example of the second. There are cases, however, of the second that are not examples of the first, when a sensation, though not perfectly reliable, depends on the fact it indicates.

The truth of color skepticism implies that we have much less perceptual knowledge than we think we have: none of the perceptual judgments in which we ascribe a color to an object are true, no less justified. But color skepticism is far from justifying some generalized Cartesian skepticism of the senses. As far as the argument in this book is concerned, there are many features we think objects have that they really do have. That this is yellow is not a case of knowledge, but that it is round may very well be something that I know to be true.

Don't our senses sometimes deceive us? That means that they are not perfectly reliable. Does not that imply that even though sensations may frequently constitute a basis that justifies many of our perceptual beliefs, they seldom or never guarantee their truth, and thus we hardly ever have perceptual knowledge? There are two points to make in response to this argument. The first is that the second type of truth selector just mentioned does not require perfect reliability, so even if our senses are frequently deceptive, we are nevertheless capable of having a great deal of perceptual knowledge. The second point is that perfect reliability may very well be achievable in some cases. Consider the following sequence of experiences: I look at the coin; it appears round; I look at it several more times; it still looks round; I look at it in daylight and in a bright light, and it still looks round. I show it to you and you and you, and it looks round to all of you; my eyes and your eyes are healthy and are not and have never been vulnerable to illnesses that affect the perception of shape. This sequence of experiences taken as a whole may very well be perfectly reliable; it may be the case that no such sequence has ever occurred or will ever occur when the object perceived is not round. If so, then I actually know it to be round.

The example of the sequence of experiences illustrates how we actually do increase the likelihood that our perceptual judgments count as knowledge. When we look at an object under adverse circumstances, we may be in doubt about its shape or other features. We then take some of the following steps; we look again and more carefully; we move closer to obtain a better view; we improve the illumination and other conditions that increase the likelihood of achieving a veridical appearance; we consult the opinion of others; and so on. These steps increase the reliability of our sensations and tend toward perfect reliability with perceptual knowledge as their outcome. Even if perfect reliability is not in fact obtained, we may approach close enough to it to trust our senses for the purposes of action. Something short of knowledge may be sufficient for the purposes of practical life.

In earlier chapters I argued for color skepticism making use of premises derived from reflections upon color science. At the beginning of this chapter I pointed out that this appears to lead to a difficulty for the argument. Color science is a set of theories based upon experience; thus color skepticism is the outcome of an argument that relies upon experience at certain points and yet challenges the pretensions of experience to provide knowledge of color. We can now understand why this is really no difficulty at all. Let E be the set of propositions that constitute the total observational evidence for all the premises that lead to color skepticism. A large number of the members of E are perceptual judgments that have nothing to do with color at all but with shape and size and distance and so forth. There is nothing in color skepticism which leads us to doubt their truth. Consider now just the subset of E, call it E*, that consists of propositions that ascribe a color to an object. E* will consist of all the color reports made by scientists and subjects that are used to support any of the theories that make up color science. Now replace E* in E with another set of propositions which consist of the sensory judgments which describe the sensations of color which triggered each of perceptual beliefs in E*. Call this new set E#. Our new set of observation reports in which E# replaces E* is capable of supporting everything in color science compatible with color skepticism. So color skepticism does not really undermine the argument for it. We have here an example of a phenomenon in science in which a theory based upon certain evidence requires a reinterpretation of the evidence on which it was based. It is not necessary that the reinterpretation diminish its confirmatory power.

There is another difficulty mentioned at the beginning of this chapter that seems to allow an opening for a more radical skepticism than I have heretofore supported. It is the classic problem for any representative theory of perception. If our knowledge of he external world is based upon sensory evidence alone or sensory evidence plus memories of previous sensations as Hume claims, how can we be sure that the external world is as our sensations represent it to be? Perhaps as Descartes claimed in the first *Meditation* there is no way to distinguish veridical from dream experience.

The basic answer to this difficulty is to distinguish two questions that are seldom distinguished in arguments over skepticism. The first question is whether or not we can prove or establish that we have perceptual knowledge. Now if radical skepticism is right, then we cannot prove that we have perceptual knowledge. But that does not show that we do not have perceptual knowledge, only that we do not know that we have it, if we do. We may have lots of perceptual knowledge of external objects even if we cannot prove that we do. At its best, skepticism is capable of undermining our epistemic right to claim that we have perceptual knowledge. But Cartesian arguments fail to show that we do not actually have it.

Can radical skepticism actually succeed in this more limited task of showing that we do not know that we know? Even this is doubtful. After all, we have lots of reasons for thinking that the conditions for the possession of knowledge are sometimes satisfied. Don't I know, for example, that the stove is hot when I touch it? Here is the stove; I see it;

my finger is in contact with it; I have this sensation which reliability indicates the presence of heat. What more do I need?

The usual reply of the skeptic is that my use of this information to show that I know that the stove is hot is not legitimate. If my only access to the external world is via my sensations, then I am only entitled to use pure sensory judgments as premises in my argument. I am not entitled to bring information about external objects into the picture as premises.

But this reply of the skeptic assumes that we can establish the notion of a pure sensory judgment without presupposing any information about the external world. It assumes that we can take the subjective turn by pure reflection upon experience without making use of our beliefs and knowledge about material objects. However, we earlier noted that the subjectivity of the content of our color and sound sensations is a conclusion based upon theories and facts about how these sensations are caused by external objects. With respect to the other sensations implicated in perception such as sensations of heat, of taste, of smell and so forth, mere reflection reveals that they possess a bodily location; it does not allow us to bracket our own bodies. The variety of considerations and arguments which lead to the subjective turn are not compatible with the generalized skepticism that Descartes wished to establish in the first of his *Meditations*. His argument there appears persuasive only because it suppresses the premises that allow the very contrast between inner and outer that it relies upon. So I do not think that the skeptic is in any position to establish that we do not know that we have perceptual knowledge of the external world.

NOTES

1. Gilbert Ryle, *The Concept of Mind* (London: Hutchinson's University Library, 1949), pp. 27-35.
2. A. J. Ayer, *The Problem of Knowledge* (New York: Penguin Books, 1984), p. 16.
3. *Ibid.* p. 17.
4. Karl R. Popper, *Objective Knowledge, an Evolutionary Approach* (Oxford: Clarendon Press, 1973), p. 163.
5. Louis Pojman objects as follows: "Being able to recall the propositions in question seems a necessary condition for knowledge." It seems to me, however, that a weaker condition is called for, namely, that one must recall where one has stored the information that one is claiming as knowledge and that one must have access to the place of storage. Perhaps my

account, influenced by Popper, constitutes a revision or extension of our original concept of knowledge that is justified by the invention of ways of storing information outside the brain.

6. This is a variation upon an example provided by Bertrand Russell in *The Problems of Philosophy* (London: Oxford University Press, 1951), pp. 131-132.

7. Edmund L. Gettier, "Is Justified True Belief Knowledge?" reprinted in A. Phillips Griffiths (ed.), *Knowledge and Belief* (London: Oxford University Press, 1967), pp. 144-146.

8. *Ibid.*, p. 145.

9. *Ibid.*

10. I employed this notion of full justification in my text *Philosophy: An Introduction to the Central Issues* (New York: Holt, Rinehart and Winston, 1985), pp. 208-210. For much the same reasons, Keith Lehrer uses the notion of complete justification in his *Theory of Knowledge* (Boulder, Colorado: Westview Press, 1990), p. 12.

11. William James, "The Will to Believe," in *The Will to Believe and Other Essays in Popular Philosophy* (New York: Longmans, Green, and Co., 1919), pp. 1-31.

12. *Ibid.*, p. 11.

13. John Locke, *An Essay concerning Human Understanding*, IV, xix, 1.

14. *Ibid.*, IV, xix, 14.

15. *Ibid.*, IV, xix, 13.

16. David Hume, *An Enquiry concerning Human Understanding*, Indianapolis: Hackett Publishing Co., 1983), p. 15.

17. *Ibid.*

18. *Ibid.*, p. 30.

INDEX

PHILOSOPHICAL STUDIES SERIES

Founded by Wilfrid S. Sellars and Keith Lehrer

1. JAY F. ROSENBERG, *Linguistic Representation,* 1974.
2. WILFRID SELLARS, *Essays in Philosophy and Its History,* 1974.
3. DICKINSON S. MILLER, *Philosophical Analysis and Human Welfare.* Selected Essays and Chapters from Six Decades. Edited with an Introduction by Lloyd D. Easton, 1975.
4. KEITH LEHRER (ed.), *Analysis and Metaphysics.* Essays in Honor of R. M. Chisholm. 1975.
5. CARL GINET, *Knowledge, Perception, and Memory,* 1975.
6. PETER H. HARE and EDWARD H. MADDEN, *Causing, Perceiving and Believing.* An Examination of the Philosophy of C. J. Ducasse, 1975.
7. HECTOR-NERI CASTAÑEDA, *Thinking and Doing.* The Philosophical Foundations of Institutions, 1975.
8. JOHN L. POLLOCK, *Subjunctive Reasoning,* 1976.
9. BRUCE AUNE, *Reason and Action,* 1977.
10. GEORGE SCHLESINGER, *Religion and Scientific Method,* 1977.
11. YIRMIAHU YOVEL (ed.), *Philosophy of History and Action.* Papers presented at the first Jerusalem Philosophical Encounter, December 1974, 1978.
12. JOSEPH C. PITT, *The Philosophy of Wilfrid Sellars: Queries and Extensions,* 1978.
13. ALVIN I. GOLDMAN and JAEGWON KIM, *Values and Morals.* Essays in Honor of William Frankena, Charles Stevenson, and Richard Brandt, 1978.
14. MICHAEL J. LOUX, *Substance and Attribute.* A Study in Ontology, 1978.
15. ERNEST SOSA (ed.), *The Philosophy of Nicholas Rescher: Discussion and Replies,* 1979.
16. JEFFRIE G. MURPHY, *Retribution, Justice, and Therapy.* Essays in the Philosophy of Law, 1979.
17. GEORGE S. PAPPAS, *Justification and Knowledge: New Studies in Epistemology,* 1979.
18. JAMES W. CORNMAN, *Skepticism, Justification, and Explanation,* 1980.
19. PETER VAN INWAGEN, *Time and Cause.* Essays presented to Richard Taylor, 1980.
20. DONALD NUTE, *Topics in Conditional Logic,* 1980.
21. RISTO HILPINEN (ed.), *Rationality in Science,* 1980.
22. GEORGES DICKER, *Perceptual Knowledge,* 1980.

23. JAY F. ROSENBERG, *One World and Our Knowledge of It,* 1980.
24. KEITH LEHRER and CARL WAGNER, *Rational Consensus in Science and Society,* 1981.
25. DAVID O'CONNOR, *The Metaphysics of G. E. Moore,* 1982.
26. JOHN D. HODSON, *The Ethics of Legal Coercion,* 1983.
27. ROBERT J. RICHMAN, *God, Free Will, and Morality,* 1983.
28. TERENCE PENELHUM, *God and Skepticism,* 1983.
29. JAMES BOGEN and JAMES E. McGUIRE (eds.), *How Things Are, Studies in Predication and the History of Philosophy of Science,* 1985.
30. CLEMENT DORE, *Theism,* 1984.
31. THOMAS L. CARSON, *The Status of Morality,* 1984.
32. MICHAEL J. WHITE, *Agency and Integrality,* 1985.
33. DONALD F. GUSTAFSON, *Intention and Agency,* 1986.
34. PAUL K. MOSER, *Empirical Justification,* 1985.
35. FRED FELDMAN, *Doing the Best We Can,* 1986.
36. G. W. FITCH, *Naming and Believing,* 1987.
37. TERRY PENNER, *The Ascent from Nominalism.* Some Existence Arguments in Plato's Middle Dialogues, 1987.
38. ROBERT G. MEYERS, *The Likelihood of Knowledge,* 1988.
39. DAVID F. AUSTIN, *Philosophical Analysis.* A Defense by Example, 1988.
40. STUART SILVERS, *Rerepresentation.* Essays in the Philosophy of Mental Rerepresentation, 1988.
41. MICHAEL P. LEVINE, *Hume and the Problem of Miracles. A Solution*, 1979.
42. MELVIN DALGARNO and ERIC MATTHEWS, *The Philosophy of Thomas Reid*, 1989.
43. KENNETH R. WESTPHAL, *Hegel's Epistemological Realism.* A Study of the Aim and Method of Hegel's *Phenomenology of Spirit*, 1989.
44. JOHN W. BENDER, *The Current State of the Coherence Theory.* Critical Essays on the Epistemic Theories of Keith Lehrer and Laurence Bonjour, with Replies, 1989.
45. ROGER D. GALLIE, *Thomas Reid and 'The Way of Ideas'*, 1989.
46. J-C. SMITH (ed.), *Historical Foundations of Cognitive Science*, 1990.
47. JOHN HEIL (ed.), *Cause, Mind, and Reality.* Essays Honoring C. B. Martin, 1990.
48. MICHAEL D. ROTH and GLENN ROSS (eds.), *Doubting.* Contemporary Perspectives on Skepticism, 1990.
49. ROD BERTOLET, *What is Said.* A Theory of Indirect Speech Reports, 1990
50. BRUCE RUSSELL (ed.), *Freedom, Rights and Pornography.* A Collection of Papers by Fred R. Berger, 1990
51. KEVIN MULLIGAN (ed.), *Language, Truth and Ontology,* 1992
52. JESÚS EZQUERRO and JESÚS M. LARRAZABAL (eds.), *Cognition, Semantics and Philosophy.* Proceedings of the First International Colloquium on Cognitive Science, 1992

53. O.H. GREEN, *The Emotions*. A Philosophical Theory, 1992
54. JEFFRIE G. MURPHY, *Retribution Reconsidered.* More Essays in the Philosophy of Law, 1992
55. PHILLIP MONTAGUE, *In the Interests of Others.* An Essay in Moral Philosophy, 1992
56. J.- P. DUBUCS (ed.), *Philosophy of Probability*. 1993
57. G.S. ROSENKRANTZ, *Haecceity:* An Ontological Essay. 1993
58. C. LANDESMAN, *The Eye and the Mind.* Reflections on Perception and the Problem of Knowledge. 1993

GPSR Compliance

The European Union's (EU) General Product Safety Regulation (GPSR) is a set of rules that requires consumer products to be safe and our obligations to ensure this.

If you have any concerns about our products, you can contact us on ProductSafety@springernature.com

In case Publisher is established outside the EU, the EU authorized representative is:

Springer Nature Customer Service Center GmbH
Europaplatz 3
69115 Heidelberg, Germany

Batch number: 10824712

Printed by Printforce, the Netherlands